Mayo Clinic
Straight Talk On Arthritis

Gene Hunder, M.D.
Medical Editor in Chief

Mayo Clinic
Rochester, Minnesota

Mayo Clinic Straight Talk On Arthritis provides reliable, practical, easy-to-understand information on osteoarthritis, rheumatoid arthritis and many related disorders. Much of the information comes directly from the experience of Mayo Clinic physicians, nurses, research scientists, health educators, therapists and other health care professionals. This book supplements the advice of your personal physician, whom you should consult for individual medical problems. *Mayo Clinic Straight Talk On Arthritis* does not endorse any company or product. MAYO, MAYO CLINIC, MAYO CLINIC HEALTH INFORMATION and the Mayo triple-shield logo are marks of Mayo Foundation for Medical Education and Research.

Published by Mayo Clinic Health Information, Rochester, Minn.

Library of Congress Control Number 2005937263

ISBN-13: 978-1-893005-40-2
ISBN-10: 1-893005-40-2

Printed in the United States of America

First Edition

1 2 3 4 5 6 7 8 9 10

About arthritis

Arthritis is one of the most common health problems in the world. It's the No. 1 cause of disability in the United States. More than 45 million Americans have some form of arthritis. So if you have arthritis, you're not alone. Although a cure has yet to be found, effective treatments and other strategies are available.

This book focuses on the two most common forms of the disease — osteoarthritis and rheumatoid arthritis — but includes information useful to people with almost any form of the disease. This book provides information you can put to use today to better manage your disease. Much of this information is what Mayo Clinic doctors, nurses and therapists use in caring for their patients.

If you understand your disease and treatment options and you put this knowledge to use in daily living, you can live more productively and comfortably, and you'll be able to communicate more effectively with your doctor and other health care professionals.

About Mayo Clinic

Mayo Clinic evolved from the frontier practice of Dr. William Worrall Mayo, and the partnership of his two sons, William J. and Charles H. Mayo, in the early 1900s. Pressed by the demands of their busy practice in Rochester, Minn., the Mayo brothers invited other physicians to join them, pioneering the private group practice of medicine. Today, with more than 2,000 physicians and scientists at its three major locations in Rochester, Minn., Jacksonville, Fla., and Scottsdale, Ariz., Mayo Clinic is dedicated to providing comprehensive diagnoses, accurate answers and effective treatments.

With this depth of medical knowledge, experience and expertise, Mayo Clinic occupies an unparalleled position as a health information resource. Since 1983, Mayo Clinic has published reliable health information for millions of consumers through award-winning newsletters, books and online services. Revenue from the publishing activities supports Mayo Clinic programs, including medical education and research.

Editorial staff

Medical Editor in Chief
Gene Hunder, M.D.

Managing Editor
Richard Dietman

Publisher
Sara Gilliland

Editor in Chief, Books and Newsletters
Christopher Frye

Research Manager
Deirdre Herman

Research Librarians
Anthony Cook
Dana Gerberi
Michelle Hewlett

Proofreading
Miranda Attlesey
Mary Duerson
Louise Filipic
Donna Hanson

Contributing Writers
Lee Engfer
Kelly Kershner

Photography
Joseph Kane
Richard Madsen

Creative Director
Daniel Brevick

Art Director
Paul Krause

Illustration
Michael King
Kent McDaniel
Christopher Srnka

Indexing
Larry Harrison

Administrative Assistant
Terri Zanto-Strausbauch

Contributing editors and reviewers

Brent Bauer, M.D.
Robert Beckenbaugh, M.D.
Lisa Buss, R.Ph.
April Chang-Miller, M.D.
Robert Cofield, M.D.
Mary Jurisson, M.D.
Susan Lepore, O.T.R.
Nisha Manek, M.D.

Thomas Mason, M.D.
Eric Matteson, M.D.
Jennifer K. Nelson, R.D.
Terry Oh, M.D.
Thomas Osborn, M.D.
John Postier, P.T.
Karen Wallevand

Preface

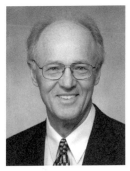

*M*ayo Clinic Straight Talk On Arthritis was prepared to help you take control of your arthritis. This book contains information about the latest arthritis drugs, including biologic agents, as well as new details about surgical procedures and places to get support. An extensive glossary is included to help explain terms with which you may be unfamiliar, as well as a chapter on complementary and alternative medicine.

Along with this information, there are tips on managing your arthritis, including protecting your joints, exercise, pain control, diet and, equally important, how to maintain a positive attitude. In addition, you'll find descriptions of a number of important but less well-known forms of arthritis.

You'll also find information on potential new treatments of arthritis. There are practical tips on traveling with arthritis and on coping with it on the job. This book concludes with a chapter that lists and describes other reliable sources of information on arthritis, including helpful recommendations for evaluating health information you find on the Web.

Mayo Clinic doctors who specialize in arthritis reviewed each chapter of this book for accuracy. They were assisted by Mayo specialists in orthopedic surgery, physical therapy, psychiatry, occupational therapy, nutrition and pain management.

We can't promise a cure for arthritis, but we can tell you that your disease doesn't have to defeat you. Arthritis can be a disabling disease. Most often it isn't.

If you consistently apply the information in this book to your daily living, you can live more productively and comfortably.

That's our commitment to you.

Gene Hunder, M.D.
Medical Editor in Chief

Contents

Part 2: Treating arthritis   77

Part 1

Understanding arthritis

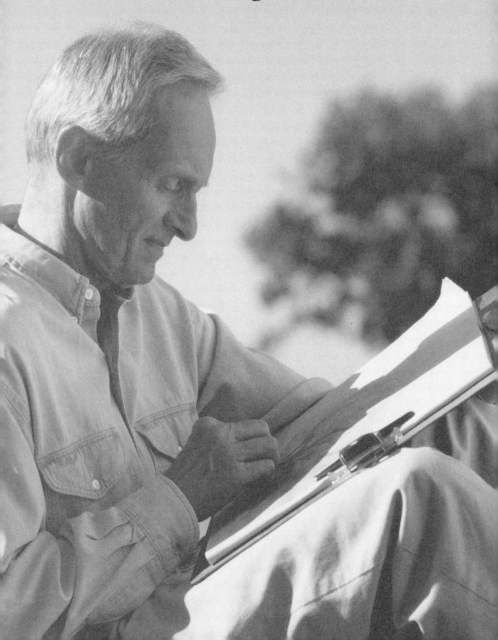

Chapter 1

Arthritis — Common and complex

W hen your joints are working smoothly, it's easy to take them for granted. But when they begin to ache, you notice. If you've experienced pain, stiffness, swelling and difficulty moving because of arthritis, you're not alone.

Arthritis is one of the most common conditions in the United States and is the leading cause of disability. One-fourth of U.S. adults report ongoing pain or stiffness in their joints, and more than 45 million Americans have been diagnosed with some form of arthritis. The costs for medical care and lost productivity amount to more than $80 billion annually. As the population ages, the number of people with arthritis is expected to increase. By 2020, an estimated 60 million people will have the disease.

Arthritis refers to diseases that affect the joints. These diseases can result in joint pain or stiffness, damage to the structure of a joint or loss of joint function. The word *arthritis* is a blend of the Greek words *arthron,* for "joint," and *itis,* for "inflammation." So arthritis literally means "joint inflammation." However, as noted above, the term *arthritis* is commonly used to refer to any disease of the joints.

Normally, inflammation is the body's response to infection or injury. The chemicals released by the immune system to fight infection cause a reaction that stimulates warmth, swelling and pain.

But some diseases involve an abnormal immune system response that creates ongoing, or chronic, inflammation.

Although people often talk about arthritis as one disease, it's not. Arthritis occurs in more than 100 forms, with varying signs and symptoms. Some forms develop gradually as a result of natural wear of joints, and others appear suddenly and then disappear, recurring at a later date. Other forms are chronic and may be progressive, getting worse over time. Arthritis can vary a great deal from one person to another, even if they have the same form.

Pain with use of affected joints and stiffness after periods of rest or inactivity are probably the best known general symptoms of arthritis. But many arthritic disorders affect more than your joints. They can also affect surrounding muscles, tendons and ligaments, as well as your skin and other organs, such as lungs, heart, bowel, brain, liver and kidneys.

Although there's no cure for arthritis, current treatments are far ahead of what was available even five or 10 years ago, and promising research offers hope of even better therapies. Early and proper treatment can help prevent joint damage and mobility problems. You can also take steps to prevent or minimize the effects of arthritis. By actively managing your arthritis — and your attitude — you can enjoy a more active and pain-free life.

Who gets arthritis?

Arthritis affects people of all ages, but it's most common among older adults. It often begins after age 40, and by age 75, more than half of adults have some form of arthritis.

Women are at higher risk of many forms of arthritis than men are. Researchers believe that female hormones may play a role. These hormones may also affect the severity of arthritis symptoms.

The likelihood of having arthritis varies by race and ethnicity. Whites, blacks and Native Americans are more likely to get arthritis than are Asians and Hispanics.

People who are more than 10 pounds overweight have a higher risk of developing arthritis, especially in the knees. Excess weight

What is rheumatism?

If your grandparents had achy joints, they might have talked about the "rheumatism" in their bones. Rheumatism is an older term for pain and stiffness in the muscles and joints. Both words — rheumatism and arthritis — are often used in a general way to describe joint problems.

Arthritis is a general term for more than 100 diseases that cause pain, swelling and stiffness in the joints. The term *rheumatic disease* is even broader, referring to any disease of the bones, muscles and joints. One feature that many of these disorders share is that they limit a person's mobility.

Rheumatology is the branch of medicine devoted to arthritis and other diseases of the musculoskeletal system, which includes the bones, joints, muscles, tendons, ligaments and other connective tissues that provide the framework and support for your body. Rheumatologists are medical doctors who have additional training and experience in rheumatology and internal medicine.

In addition to treating the many forms of arthritis, rheumatologists treat other connective tissue diseases — illnesses in which a person's immune system produces antibodies against his or her own tissues. Rheumatologists also treat musculoskeletal pain disorders, including back pain, fibromyalgia and bursitis, and bone diseases such as osteoporosis.

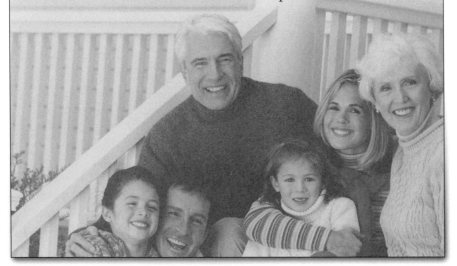

Anatomy of a joint

Joints are places in your body where two or more bones join together to form a moveable connection. The joints in your body are designed for a lifetime of service.

Bones in your joints are covered with shock-absorbing cartilage. Cartilage is a tough, smooth, slippery material that prevents bone-against-bone contact, allowing for easy movement with little friction.

Joints known as synovial joints, found in the shoulders, elbows, wrists, fingers, hips, knees, ankles and toes, are the most mobile. These joints are surrounded by a tough, fibrous capsule that attaches to bone on either side of the joint. The joint capsule helps stabilize and protect the joint. The capsule is lined with a tissue called the synovium. This thin membrane produces synovial fluid, a clear substance that nourishes the cartilage and bones and lubricates or "oils" the joint so that it can move smoothly.

Ligaments are tough cords of fibrous tissue that attach bone to bone. They help support the joint and keep it in proper alignment. Muscles and tendons also hold the joint together. Tendons — which connect muscle and bone — attach to bone just outside the capsule above or below the joint.

Bursae are small, fluid-filled sacs between muscles, or between muscles, tendons and bone. Synovial membranes line the inside of each bursa and release a lubricating fluid to cushion the joint and reduce friction.

puts more pressure on joints. A past joint injury can also increase your risk of arthritis.

What causes arthritis?

Osteoarthritis, the most common form of arthritis, involves the wearing away of the tough, lubricated cartilage that normally cushions the ends of bones in your joints. Other forms of arthritis, such

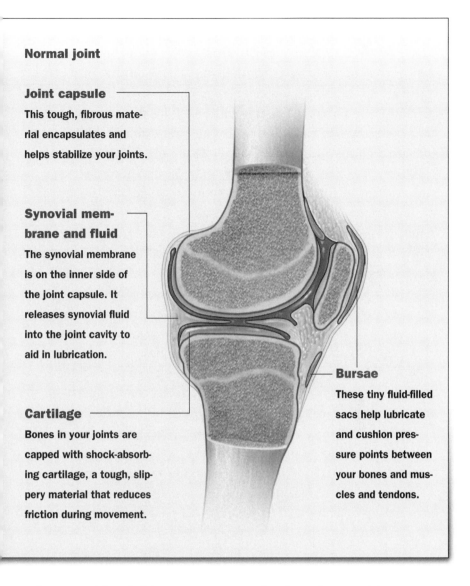

Normal joint

Joint capsule
This tough, fibrous material encapsulates and helps stabilize your joints.

Synovial membrane and fluid
The synovial membrane is on the inner side of the joint capsule. It releases synovial fluid into the joint cavity to aid in lubrication.

Cartilage
Bones in your joints are capped with shock-absorbing cartilage, a tough, slippery material that reduces friction during movement.

Bursae
These tiny fluid-filled sacs help lubricate and cushion pressure points between your bones and muscles and tendons.

as rheumatoid arthritis, occur as a result of an abnormal immune system response that causes inflammation of the lining of the joints.

Most of the underlying causes of arthritis are unclear. Researchers believe that it results from an interplay of multiple factors, both genetic and environmental. Osteoarthritis used to be thought of as a normal consequence of aging, but some people never develop the condition. Aging and wear and tear on joints over time do contribute to osteoarthritis, but other factors also play a role.

Can arthritis be prevented?

Many of the risk factors for arthritis, such as your inherited genes, your age and your gender, aren't in your control. But there are some things you can do to help lower your risk of arthritis. Even if you're beginning to feel the pain of arthritis, you can influence the severity of your symptoms and how the disease affects you.

One of the best ways to prevent pain and joint damage is to see a doctor as soon as you have symptoms such as joint pain, stiffness or swelling. Early diagnosis and proper treatment can help prevent much of the damage arthritis can bring.

To help prevent arthritis or minimize its effects, follow these guidelines:

- **Maintain a healthy weight.** Being overweight or obese increases your chance of getting osteoarthritis. And if you do have arthritis, the pressure on your joints from excess pounds can make your symptoms worse.
- **Avoid joint injuries.** Injuries to joints can lead to arthritis. When participating in physical activities, make sure to warm up to prepare your body for exercise and stretch appropriately afterward.
- **Treat injuries promptly.** If you do have an injury, tend to it properly and immediately. This will help the injury heal correctly and limit possible joint damage down the road.
- **Stay physically active.** Exercise keeps your joints flexible and your muscles strong. Aerobic exercise, such as walking, helps you maintain flexibility. Strength training, such as weightlifting, strengthens the muscles around your joints, which helps protect joints.
- **Use good body mechanics to avoid joint stress.** Use your large joints and largest muscles for tasks such as lifting. Don't lift or move things that are too heavy for you. Perform daily tasks with proper body mechanics to avoid overloading your joints.
- **Avoid cigarette smoking.** Many studies suggest that smoking increases the risk of developing rheumatoid arthritis.

Quitting smoking may prevent the development of this form of arthritis.

- **Pay attention to what you eat.** There's no magic diet or food that can prevent arthritis. But some evidence suggests that people whose diets are high in olive oil may have less chance of developing rheumatoid arthritis. Olive oil is a good source of monounsaturated fatty acids and may have anti-inflammatory effects. However, little research has been done specifically on the possible benefits of olive oil for people with arthritis. Vitamin D may also help protect against rheumatoid arthritis and osteoarthritis. Dietary sources of vitamin D include eggs and fortified breads, cereals and milk. Brief exposure to sunlight is the easiest way to get vitamin D.

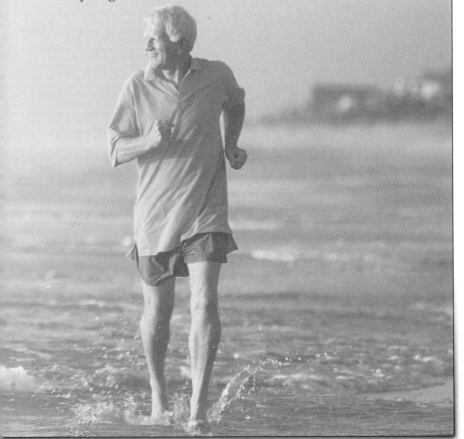

Heredity and genetic makeup can influence whether or not you get arthritis. For example, scientists have identified specific genes that are linked to an increased risk of developing rheumatoid arthritis. Studies have also shown that genetic factors contribute to some cases of osteoarthritis. But even people who are genetically predisposed to develop arthritis won't necessarily do so. Other factors are involved in triggering the disease.

Other possible contributing factors may include infectious agents such as viruses, bacteria, fungi or parasites, toxic materials, or substances in food, water or air that could trigger the onset of arthritis. An imbalance of certain hormones or enzymes could possibly play a role. Physical trauma, such as an ankle sprain or a knee injury, can set the stage for osteoarthritis and other types of arthritis. Lack of physical activity, excess weight and joint defects such as bowlegs can also lead to arthritis. Stress or other forms of emotional trauma can worsen symptoms.

Common forms of arthritis

The vast majority of people with arthritis have one of two forms — osteoarthritis or rheumatoid arthritis. Osteoarthritis is the most common type. Rheumatoid arthritis, the other main type, affects one-tenth as many people but can be much more debilitating. Find more on rheumatoid arthritis in Chapter 3.

All forms of arthritis can cause some common symptoms, such as joint pain or tenderness, stiffness, difficulty moving and swelling around joints. In addition, other musculoskeletal conditions can cause joint discomfort. Although new tests make it easier to diagnose arthritis, there still aren't definitive lab or imaging tests that can pinpoint the cause of symptoms in every case.

For these reasons, diagnosing arthritis can be a challenge. Your doctor will rely on your description of symptoms and other information, as well as a physical exam. These are key to early diagnosis and treatment. A series of visits over time may be necessary before your doctor determines the exact cause of your signs and symptoms.

When to call a doctor

Most often arthritis isn't a medical emergency. But treatment is often more effective when symptoms are caught early. In addition, some symptoms require immediate attention.

If you have arthritis symptoms that you know are from overdoing it and they disappear in a few days, you probably don't need to call your doctor. But call your doctor if:

- New pain develops or you have persistent symptoms lasting more than several days
- You have joint pain accompanied by fever, rash, headache or weight loss
- You have severe or worsening pain in one or a few joints
- You have numbness or pain in your hands or legs or pain that radiates from your neck or low back
- You experience joint injury or trauma

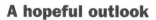

A hopeful outlook

Despite aches and pains and the joint problems that arthritis causes, most people with arthritis get on with their lives and control their symptoms successfully. The two most common forms of arthritis, osteoarthritis and rheumatoid arthritis, aren't ordinarily life-threatening and respond well to medical treatments and self-care.

Start by learning as much as you can about your type of arthritis, your treatment options and, most importantly, the steps you can take to control your arthritis in partnership with your physician. The following chapters in this book will give you information as well as tools and strategies for living with a chronic disease.

Armed with this information and a positive attitude, you can move forward, adjusting your lifestyle without compromising your happiness and fulfillment.

Chapter 2

Osteoarthritis, localized musculoskeletal conditions and osteoporosis

Osteoarthritis is the most common form of arthritis, especially in older adults. There are also some other conditions, including back pain, bursitis and tendinitis, that at least initially may be confused with osteoarthritis. In this chapter, you'll learn about osteoarthritis, its signs and symptoms and how it's diagnosed and treated. And you'll find information on related conditions.

Osteoarthritis

If you have osteoarthritis, you might be stiff and achy when you get out of bed every morning — but feel less creaky by the time you finish your first cup of coffee. Your fingers may be stiff, with bony lumps, making it hard to hold a pen or open a jar. After a game of tennis or a jog in the park, your knees may hurt.

Osteoarthritis, sometimes called degenerative arthritis or degenerative joint disease, affects 21 million Americans. The disease is more common in women than in men. Osteoarthritis may affect any joint in your body, but it most often occurs in the hands, knees, hips and back. Initially it tends to affect only one joint. But if your hands are affected, multiple finger joints may become arthritic.

With osteoarthritis, the problem lies in the cartilage that cushions the ends of bones in your joints. Over time, the cartilage wears away and its smooth surface roughens. At this point many people have intermittent pain in the affected joint, especially with strenuous use. Eventually, if the cartilage wears down completely, you may be left with bone rubbing on bone, and the ends of your bones become damaged. This is usually painful in nearly everyone with osteoarthritis.

Your body attempts to repair the damage, but the repairs are usually inadequate, resulting instead in growth of new bone, or spurs, along the sides of the existing bone. This produces prominent lumps, which most often occur with osteoarthritis of the hands and feet. The pain and tenderness over the bony lumps may be most marked early in the course of the disease and less noticeable later on. If the cartilage in a joint is severely damaged, the synovium may become inflamed. This low-grade inflammation, called synovitis, can cause episodes of joint swelling.

Some scientists believe the cartilage damage may be due to an imbalance of enzymes released from the cartilage cells or from the lining of the joint. When balanced, these enzymes allow for the natural breakdown and regeneration of cartilage. But too much of the enzymes can cause the joint cartilage to break down faster than it's rebuilt. The exact cause of this enzyme imbalance is unclear.

Early changes to the cartilage and bone don't always result in pain or other symptoms, however. Many older adults have osteoarthritis but don't know it until their doctor sees it on a routine X-ray. In some studies, half or more of people whose X-rays show evidence of osteoarthritis don't have any symptoms.

Osteoarthritis most often develops after age 40 — it's relatively rare among young people unless they have a joint injury. Those who are affected often have a family history of the disease. Although an active lifestyle may slow the process, almost everyone over age 65 has some joint damage and mild symptoms of osteoarthritis. Men usually develop symptoms before age 55, while women typically don't have symptoms until after that age.

Severe injury to one or more joints at an early age may lead to osteoarthritis years later. Similarly, excessive stressful use of joints

Joint changes in osteoarthritis

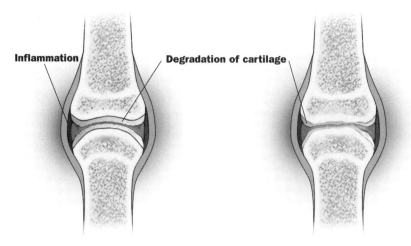

A. The first signs of osteoarthritis are microscopic pits and fissures on the cartilage surface, which are usually accompanied by a mild inflammatory reaction.

B. As the cartilage covering the surfaces of the bones of the joint is worn completely through, the contours of the joint are changed and patches of exposed bone appear.

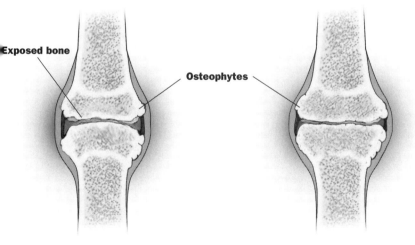

C. The subsurface bone thickens and osteophytes (spurs) develop. Use of the joint causes pain.

D. In advanced stages, the joint space may disappear and ligaments loosen, causing further joint instability. The irregular joint surfaces can cause marked limitation of motion.

over years, such as in a job that requires repeated knee bending, may cause osteoarthritis in those joints later on. If certain activities cause pain in one or more joints, avoid those activities until you've had the painful area examined by a doctor.

Being overweight also increases your risk of developing osteoarthritis, especially in the hips and knees. In one study, women who were heaviest were twice as likely to get osteoarthritis and had three times the risk for knee osteoarthritis. Losing excess weight can help you reduce your risk. (See Chapter 12 for information on weight management.)

Signs and symptoms

Osteoarthritis usually develops slowly. At first many people notice pain and stiffness only after a bout of strenuous activity or when first getting up in the morning. The morning stiffness of osteoarthritis usually passes in less than 30 minutes, a phenomenon called gelling.

If you have osteoarthritis, you may experience:

- Pain or tenderness in a joint during or after use, or after a period of inactivity

Normal spine   **Osteoarthritic spine**

Disk

Nerve

Vertebra

Bone spur

Narrowed disk

Elastic structures called disks cushion the vertebrae in a normal spine, keeping the spine flexible. In osteoarthritis, disks may narrow and bone spurs form. Pain and stiffness may occur where bone surfaces rub together, and the spine becomes less flexible.

- Discomfort in a joint before or during a change in the weather
- Swelling and stiffness in a joint, particularly after using it
- Bony lumps on the middle or end joints of your fingers or the base of your thumb
- Loss of flexibility of a joint

Osteoarthritis commonly occurs in the neck or back. The disks between the vertebrae of your spine are made of cartilage. These disks can wear down. When this happens, the spaces between the bones narrow. Bony outgrowths, called spurs (osteophytes), may form. When bone surfaces rub together, the joint and areas around the cartilage become inflamed, causing stiffness and pain.

Gradually, your spine stiffens and loses flexibility. If several disks are involved, you may notice a loss of height.

Spinal stenosis is a condition associated with osteoarthritis of the spine. Spinal stenosis occurs when degenerating disks and bone spurs bulge into the spinal canal and press on the spinal cord or

X-ray image of advanced osteoarthritis of the spine. Note misaligned vertebrae and uneven spaces between individual vertebra.

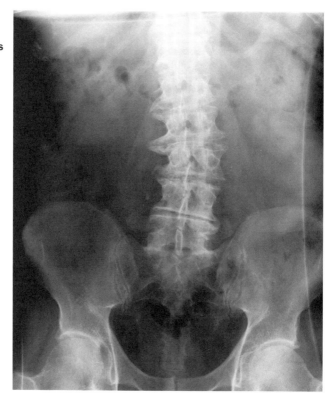

X-ray image of knees affected by osteo-arthritis. Note uneven spaces and actual points of contact between thigh bone (femur) and shin bone (tibia) on the inside of the joints.

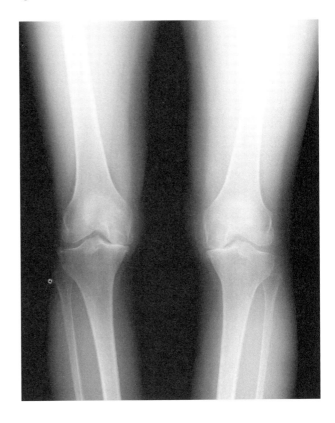

nerve roots where they exit the spine between the vertebrae. This is commonly referred to as pinched nerves. You may feel pain in your neck, shoulders, arms, lower back or even legs. (Spinal stenosis is discussed in more detail on pages 25-27.)

Osteoarthritis also frequently affects the weight-bearing joints of the hips, knees and feet. You may have chronic pain or pain that you feel when you stand, walk, get up from a chair or go up stairs. Your knee may be swollen and you may feel a grating or "catching" sensation when you move it. This sometimes even makes a sound.

In the feet, the joint where the big toe attaches to the foot is the most frequent location of osteoarthritis. The joint becomes larger with bony swelling and less flexible. You may find it uncomfortable to wear shoes and painful to walk.

In the hands, the fingertip (distal) joints and those in the middle of the fingers tend to be affected most often by osteoarthritis. The joint at the base of the thumb also is a common site for osteoarthri-tis to develop. These joints may be painful or tender and show

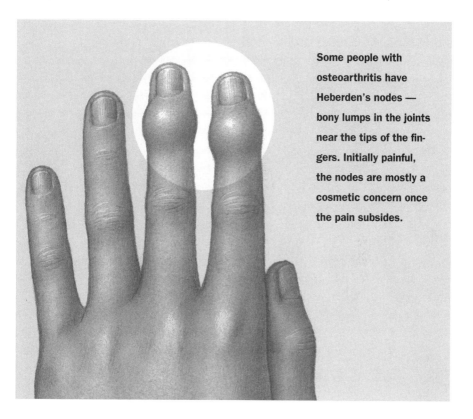

Some people with osteoarthritis have Heberden's nodes — bony lumps in the joints near the tips of the fingers. Initially painful, the nodes are mostly a cosmetic concern once the pain subsides.

some redness or swelling, especially early on. Eventually, the acute discomfort lessens. Bony growths (spurs) may form. Growths in the distal joints are called Heberden's nodes, while spurs that grow in the middle joints are called Bouchard's nodes.

Osteoarthritis often affects joints on just one side of the body, especially early in its course. Gradually, joints on the opposite side of your body may become involved as well.

The pain of early osteoarthritis often tends to fade within a year, but it can return if you overuse the affected joint. Still, unless multiple joints are involved, the effects of osteoarthritis are likely to be mild. Keeping fit helps prevent problems.

Diagnosing osteoarthritis

If you think you may have osteoarthritis, schedule an appointment with your doctor. The diagnosis is usually based on your symptoms and medical history and a physical examination.

Your doctor may ask about your joint symptoms, such as pain,

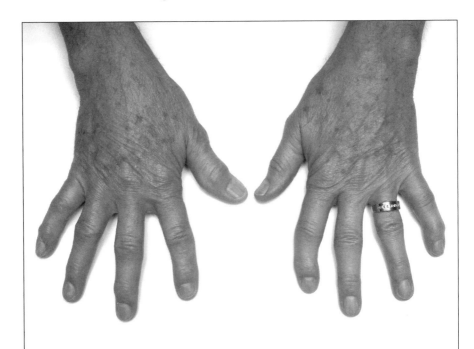

These hands of a person with osteoarthritis show how finger joints may become misaligned and lumpy over time.

swelling or stiffness. The nature of the joint pain and the specific joints affected can help distinguish between different forms of arthritis. Your doctor may also want to know whether your symptoms started gradually or suddenly, how they've changed over time and how they're affected by activity. For example, mild morning stiffness is common in osteoarthritis and usually gets better after a few minutes of activity. In contrast, morning stiffness that lasts for hours is more likely to be a symptom of rheumatoid arthritis or another inflammatory disorder.

Your doctor may also ask about any other symptoms you have, such as fever, fatigue or skin problems. It's important to note any events that occurred just before your symptoms began and whether you have a family history of arthritis.

During the physical exam, the doctor will look at your joints for swelling and bony enlargements and listen and feel for a crunching or grating sensation (crepitation) as evidence of irregularities in the surfaces of the joint cartilage. The doctor will also move your joints

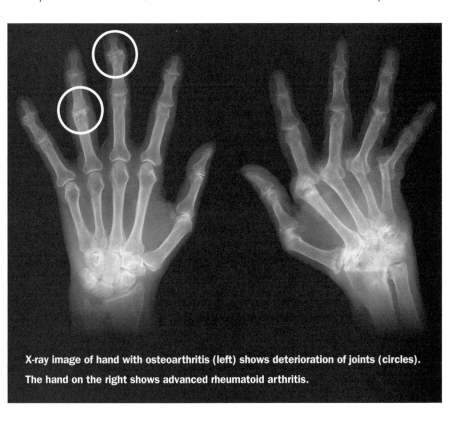

X-ray image of hand with osteoarthritis (left) shows deterioration of joints (circles). The hand on the right shows advanced rheumatoid arthritis.

through their range of motion to detect pain in certain positions or limitation of motion.

Your doctor may recommend imaging studies to confirm the diagnosis, rule out other causes of pain and determine the extent of joint damage. But X-ray findings may be normal early on, because initial changes in the cartilage occur before they can be seen on X-rays. Later, bone spurs and wearing away of cartilage may be seen in X-rays of the affected joint. Magnetic resonance imaging (MRI) can show beginning changes in joints, but this test may not be needed.

There is no blood test for osteoarthritis, but doctors sometimes use various blood tests to help rule out rheumatoid and other forms of arthritis. Information on blood tests for arthritis is found on pages 46-47.

Remember, the presence of osteoarthritis does not in itself indicate a serious problem. Many people have no symptoms or disability from their arthritis. They don't even realize that they have osteoarthritis and experience little if any discomfort.

Arthritis and the weather

Do you ever feel like a human barometer? Many people with arthritis and other musculoskeletal conditions are sensitive to changes in the weather. When the temperature goes up or down or the barometric pressure shifts, their symptoms get worse.

This phenomenon is common but not well understood. Whatever the cause, a sensitivity to weather doesn't appear to influence the course of arthritis. If your symptoms are exacerbated by weather changes, you might want to temporarily increase your use of pain relievers.

Another temperature-related condition that affects some people with arthritic disorders is called Raynaud's phenomenon. In response to cold temperatures (or strong emotions), spasm of blood vessels in your hands and feet cause color changes in your skin. Your fingers or toes turn white or blue and then red. You may also feel tingling, numbness or pain in the affected areas.

Treatment

While there's no known cure for osteoarthritis, treatments can help to reduce pain and maintain joint movement. Your doctor may recommend a combination of treatments that may include medications, exercise, self-care, physical and occupational therapy, and joint protection. In some cases, surgical procedures may be necessary.

You can learn more about treatments for osteoarthritis in later chapters of this book, which deal with self-care techniques, medications, alternative treatments, surgery and new therapies on the horizon.

Other musculoskeletal conditions

Osteoarthritis is just one of many conditions that affect your musculoskeletal system. Joint pain may stem from problems in the joint itself — or nearby bones, ligaments, tendons, muscles, nerves and other tissues. Symptoms of arthritis and other musculoskeletal conditions often overlap, which can make diagnosis a challenge.

A number of musculoskeletal conditions are associated with arthritis — either by causing joint pain or stiffness, or by occurring along with or stemming from arthritis. Following are some common conditions related to arthritis.

Back pain

Back pain is one of the most common maladies. Four out of five adults experience at least one bout of back pain at some point in life. Most back pain isn't long-term — it lasts just a few days to a few weeks.

The most common site for back pain is the lower back because it bears the most weight and stress. Low back pain can have many causes, from poor posture to a cancerous growth. The most common cause is an injury to a muscle or a ligament (strain). These injuries usually result from exerting too much force on your back or overusing it in repetitious tasks. An injured muscle may "knot up" in a spasm.

Other common causes of back pain include osteoarthritis, a herniated (ruptured) disk, osteoporosis (see page 32) and fibromyalgia (see page 30). Less common causes include spinal stenosis (see page 25) and ankylosing spondylitis (see page 58). Other forms of arthritis can also cause back pain.

Diagnosis. Most back pain disappears with home treatment and self-care. Although it may take a few weeks before back pain goes away completely, you should feel some improvement within the first 72 hours. If not, see your doctor. Also see your doctor if you're older than age 50, have a history of back pain or cancer or your back pain:

- Feels constant or intense, especially at night
- Spreads down one or both legs
- Causes weakness, numbness or tingling in one or both legs
- Causes new bowel or bladder problems
- Is associated with abdominal pain or throbbing
- Is the result of a fall or blow to your back
- Is accompanied by unexplained weight loss

Your doctor will examine your back and assess your ability to sit, stand, walk and lift your legs. Diagnostic tests aren't usually

Questions your doctor may ask

To diagnose any form of arthritis, a doctor relies heavily on your description of signs and symptoms and other relevant information. It's a good idea to make a list of your signs and symptoms and when and where they occur. Keeping a pain record or diary for two weeks can help your doctor make a diagnosis. Keep track of the intensity of your pain, how long it lasts, what it feels like and whether anything makes it better or worse.

Following are some questions you may be asked about your symptoms:

- How many joints are affected? Which joints are painful?
- Do the same joints on both sides of your body hurt at the same time, or is the pain just on one side?
- Has the pain moved from one joint to another?
- Did pain start in just one joint and then progress to include others? How quickly did this happen?
- Did your symptoms start gradually or all at once? Have they gotten worse over time or stayed about the same?
- Do you have stiffness in the morning or after a period of inactivity, such as when watching TV? How long does morning stiffness last?
- What time of day is the pain most severe?
- If you have pain in your hands, which joints hurt the most?
- Have you had times of feeling weak and uncomfortable all over? Have you been unusually tired?
- Does anything make your pain better or worse?
- Does pain or difficulty moving interfere with your work, sleep or daily activities?
- Do you have any other symptoms besides joint problems?
- Does arthritis or rheumatic disease run in your family?
- Before your symptoms first appeared, did you have a viral or bacterial illness, injury, vaccination or new medication?

needed to confirm the cause of back pain. But if your doctor suspects a tumor, fracture, infection or other serious problem, he or she may order imaging tests, such as X-rays, magnetic resonance imaging (MRI), computerized tomography (CT) or bone scans. An electromyography (EMG) test can help detect nerve compression caused by spinal stenosis.

Treatment. Many back problems respond to home treatments such as anti-inflammatory medication, ice, heat or gentle massage. Studies show that most cases of back pain improve in a matter of weeks, regardless of the type of treatment used. If your pain hasn't resolved within four weeks, your doctor may suggest muscle relaxants, electrical stimulation or physical therapy.

Although back pain is more common as you get older, it's not inevitable. You can prevent many back problems by doing exercises that strengthen the muscles that support your back and practicing good posture and work habits that protect your back.

Spinal stenosis

Spinal stenosis (stuh-NO-sis) is a narrowing of an area in your spinal canal that can cause compression of your spinal cord and nerve roots. The spinal cord is a bundle of nerves and nerve cells that extends the length of your spine. The cord is housed inside a channel, or canal, within the vertebrae, the bones of the spine. The nerves that branch off from the spinal cord provide communication between your brain and the rest of your body.

Spinal stenosis puts pressure on the spinal cord or on the roots of the nerves that branch out from the spinal cord. This pressure can result in a wide range of problems, including pain, cramping or numbness in your legs, back, neck, shoulders or arms.

Between 250,000 and 500,000 Americans have spinal stenosis. It typically affects adults over age 50. Most often, the spinal narrowing results from osteoarthritis, but injuries, other diseases and even tumors can also lead to the condition.

As the cartilage covering the surfaces of the joints in your spine wears away from osteoarthritis, the disks between the vertebrae may become worn and spaces between vertebrae may narrow. Bony outgrowths (spurs) may develop. These changes can cause

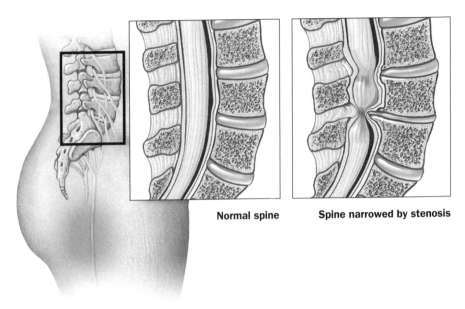

Normal spine   **Spine narrowed by stenosis**

Spinal stenosis may result when vertebrae become worn and narrowed by osteoarthritis. The narrowing can put pressure on your spinal cord, causing pain, numbness and tingling in your hips, buttocks and legs.

vertebrae and soft tissue to move inward into the spinal canal (see image above).

Spinal narrowing doesn't always cause problems. But if the narrowed areas put pressure on the spinal cord or the base of the spinal nerves, you're likely to develop signs and symptoms. An inflammatory response may also play a role in the development of symptoms.

Signs and symptoms. These often start gradually and worsen over time. You may first notice an ache in your buttock, thigh and calf when you walk and stand. Other symptoms include:

- Pain that starts in your hip or buttocks and radiates downward along the path of the sciatic nerve, which extends down the back of each leg
- Numbness, tingling or cramping of your legs
- Difficulty standing or walking
- Low back pain
- Pain in the neck and shoulders
- Loss of balance
- Bowel and bladder problems

The pain of spinal stenosis usually improves if you lean forward, crouch or sit down. You likely notice the pain more when you walk downhill. This is different from leg pain that occurs as a result of poor circulation, which is usually worse when you walk uphill and improves when you stop walking and stand still.

Diagnosis. Spinal stenosis can be difficult to diagnose because leg pain is often the main symptom. In addition to a physical exam, you're also likely to have imaging tests, such as a spinal X-ray, MRI, CT (computerized tomography) scan or others.

Treatment. Many people with spinal stenosis find effective relief with pain relievers or NSAIDs, rest, physical therapy, exercise and other conservative treatments. If you have intolerable pain that interferes with your ability to walk or do other activities, progressive weakness in your legs, or reduced control of your bladder or bowel, your doctor may recommend a surgical procedure to relieve pressure on the spinal cord or nerves and maintain the strength and integrity of your spine.

Bursitis

Whether you're at work or play, if you overuse or repetitively stress the area around your body's joints, you may eventually develop bursitis — a painful inflammation of a bursa. A bursa is a small, fluid-filled sac that lubricates and cushions pressure points between your bones and the tendons and muscles near your joints. You have more than 150 bursae in your body, allowing your joints to move with ease.

Bursitis occurs when one of the bursae becomes inflamed. When this happens, movement or pressure in the area is painful. Bursitis often affects the areas around the joints in your shoulders, elbows or hips. But you can also have bursitis in your knee, heel and even in the base of your big toe.

Common causes of bursitis are overuse, stress or injury to a joint. For example, if you spend a lot of time kneeling, the pressure could cause a bursa in front of your kneecap to become inflamed. Swinging a racket or golf club or throwing a ball repeatedly can affect a bursa in your elbow or shoulder. Bursitis may also result from an infection or gout. Many times, the cause is unknown.

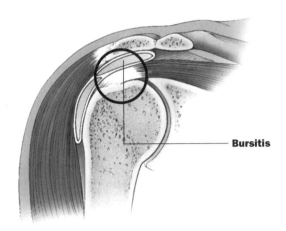

Bursitis

Bursitis is the inflammation or irritation of a bursa, a sac-like structure that helps cushion a joint. Bursitis — shown here in the shoulder — may occur with various forms of arthritis.

Because bursae are near joints, people sometimes mistake the pain of bursitis for arthritis. Some forms of arthritis can also lead to bursitis.

Signs and symptoms. If you have bursitis, you may feel an ache or tenderness around your elbow, hip, knee, shoulder, big toe or another joint. The joint may be stiff and difficult to move. The pain worsens with movement. If the inflamed bursa is near the skin, the area around it may be red, swollen and warm to the touch.

Bursitis of the hip doesn't cause any visible swelling or skin redness because the joint's bursae are located beneath bulky muscles. In this type of bursitis, pain is primarily over the greater trochanter, a portion of your thighbone that juts out just below where the bone joins the hip.

Diagnosis. Bursitis can often be diagnosed with a careful physical exam. Your doctor may be able to identify specific areas of tenderness. To help rule out other possible causes of the discomfort, you may have an X-ray, MRI or ultrasound.

Treatment. Bursitis pain usually goes away within a week or so with home treatment, including resting the affected area, applying ice to reduce swelling, and taking nonsteroidal anti-inflammatory drugs to relieve pain and reduce inflammation. Preventing future flare-ups is important to avoid having bursitis become a chronic problem. Prevention includes joint protection, avoidance of repetitive activities, and stretching and strengthening the area.

Tendinitis

Tendons are thick, fibrous cords that attach muscles to bones and other structures. Tendinitis is traditionally defined as inflammation of the tendons, though in many cases the degree of inflammation may actually be minimal. With aging and stressful use, the tendons may become worn and frayed with partial or sometimes complete tears.

The condition causes pain and tenderness just outside a joint over the involved tendon, most often around your shoulders, elbows and knees. Some common names for tendinitis are tennis elbow, golfer's elbow, pitcher's shoulder, swimmer's shoulder and jumper's knee. Pain may also occur in the groin or above your heel, in the Achilles tendon.

The most common cause of tendinitis is injury or overuse during work or play. Professional athletes and weekend warriors alike are

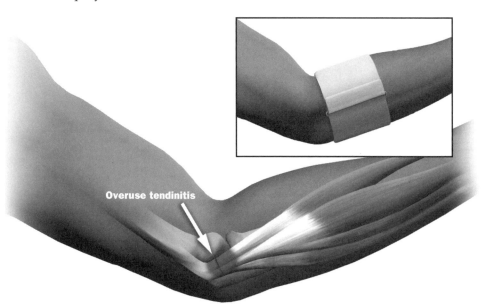

Overuse tendinitis

The pain of tendinitis is usually caused by inflammation or tiny tears (micro tears) in a tendon that joins muscle and bone. Tendinitis may result from overuse, the wear and tear of aging, or arthritis. Some people get relief from the pain of tendinitis by using an elastic bandage near the point of the inflammation.

susceptible. Tendinitis may also develop in conjunction with rheumatoid arthritis and other inflammatory rheumatic diseases. The risk of developing tendinitis increases with age, as muscles and tendons lose their elasticity.

Signs and symptoms. The location of the pain of tendinitis depends on which tendon is affected. For example, tennis elbow causes pain on the outer side of your forearm near your elbow when you rotate your forearm or grip an object. The pain is usually worse during activities that use the muscle attached to the involved tendon.

Diagnosis. Tendinitis often doesn't require a doctor's care. If pain interferes with your normal activities or doesn't improve after two weeks, see your doctor. To help rule out other possible problems, you may have an X-ray, MRI or ultrasound.

Treatment. Treatment usually focuses on resting the tendon to allow healing, applying ice to reduce swelling and taking pain relievers as needed. If the elbow or knee is involved, wrapping it with an elastic band may be helpful. Corticosteroid injections may also be helpful. Discomfort may disappear within a few weeks. In older adults and those who continue to use the affected area, tendinitis often heals more slowly and may become chronic. The involved tendon may even tear or rupture. Because of their similar locations in the body, bursitis and tendinitis may occur together.

Fibromyalgia

People with fibromyalgia often say they hurt all over or feel as if they always have the flu. Fibromyalgia is a condition marked by widespread aching and stiffness and fatigue. Fibromyalgia differs from arthritis in that the pain is not in the joints but in nearby tissues — your muscles, tendons and ligaments. And unlike arthritis, fibromyalgia doesn't cause inflammation — just pain.

Fibromyalgia affects an estimated 3 million to 6 million people in the United States. Approximately 80 percent to 90 percent of those affected are women. It's thought to be the most common cause of musculoskeletal pain in women between the ages of 20 and 75. Several factors may contribute to the development of fibromyalgia:

- Altered pain-processing pathways in the brain and central nervous system, leading to abnormal sensitivity to pain
- Changes in the regulation of brain chemicals called neurotransmitters
- Sleep disturbances
- Injury or infection
- Changes in muscle metabolism
- Stress or emotional trauma

Signs and symptoms. The main symptom of fibromyalgia is widespread, generalized musculoskeletal pain that lasts at least three months. The pain may be a deep ache, a burning sensation or soreness. Most people with fibromyalgia feel some degree of muscle pain all the time. It may vary depending on the time of day, activity level, the weather, lack of sleep, and stress or anxiety.

The pain of fibromyalgia is felt in many areas in the body, such as the neck, back, arms, legs and chest. These areas are often tender. One of the criteria for diagnosing the condition is abnormal pain

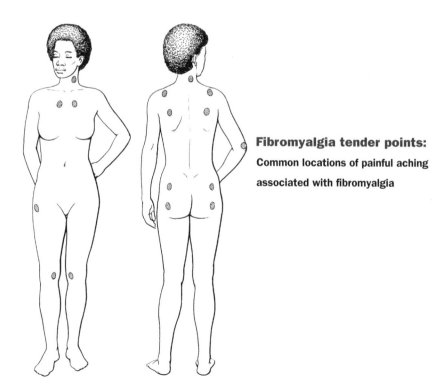

Fibromyalgia tender points:
Common locations of painful aching associated with fibromyalgia

sensitivity in a number of specific sites on the body. These areas, called tender points, are painful when pressed.

Sometimes people with fibromyalgia feel as if their joints are swollen, even though the joints aren't inflamed. Other symptoms may include:

- Chronic fatigue
- Difficulty sleeping — trouble falling asleep, waking up many times during the night or waking up unrefreshed or exhausted
- Stiffness
- Headaches and facial or jaw pain
- Digestive problems, such as abdominal pain, bloating, constipation or diarrhea
- Numbness or tingling in the hands and feet
- Depression, anxiety or mood changes
- Sensitivity to weather and temperature changes
- Sensitivity to odors, noises, bright lights and touch

Diagnosis. It's often difficult to diagnose fibromyalgia because symptoms are similar to those of other illnesses and there's no single, specific laboratory test for it. Some people have fibromyalgia along with osteoarthritis, rheumatoid arthritis or systemic lupus erythematous, which adds to the challenge of accurate diagnosis. Doctors generally diagnose fibromyalgia only after they've ruled out other conditions, which can be a lengthy process.

Treatment. Although fibromyalgia tends to stay with you, it isn't progressive or life-threatening. It doesn't damage tissues, and with treatment you can manage symptoms. Treatment often includes medications to relieve pain and improve sleep. In addition to pain relievers such as acetaminophen (Tylenol, others), medications may include nonsteroidal anti-inflammatory drugs (NSAIDs), tramadol (Ultram), antidepressants and muscle relaxants. For more information on these medications, see Chapter 8.

Cognitive behavior therapy can also be helpful, along with self-care techniques such as stress reduction and regular exercise.

Osteoporosis

Unlike osteoarthritis, which is caused by a breakdown of cartilage within joints, osteoporosis is a bone-weakening disease. It's caused

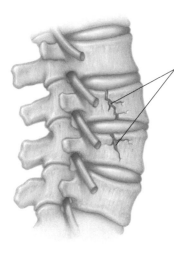

Fractures

As osteoporosis causes bone to thin and become more porous, vertebrae of the spine may become compressed and fracture, resulting in loss of height and a forward curvature of the spine.

Bones of different densities will appear differently on an X-ray image. This image of the pelvis and spine shows areas of denser bone (lighter areas) and more porous bone (darker areas). The bone affected by osteoporosis is darker.

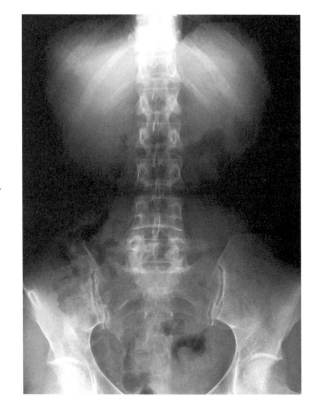

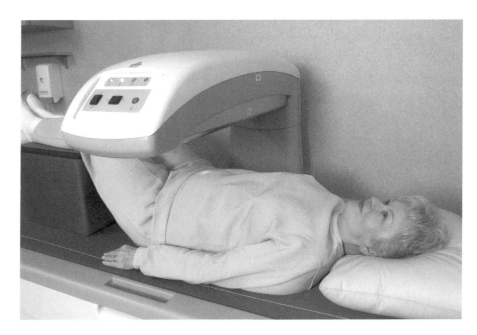

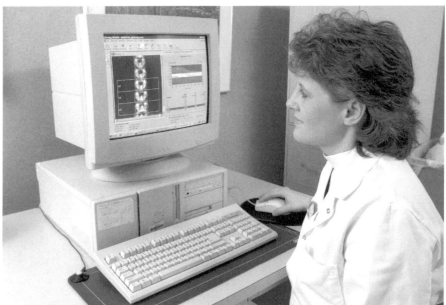

Dual energy X-ray absorptiometry (DEXA) is the most accurate procedure to screen or diagnose for osteoporosis. To have the density of your spine measured using DEXA, you lie flat on your back with your legs raised on a foam cube (top photo). The arm of the DEXA device positioned over your spine detects energy from an X-ray source located under the table. This information is transmitted to a computer (bottom photo). An image of the bone appears on the screen along with a summary table of bone density measurements.

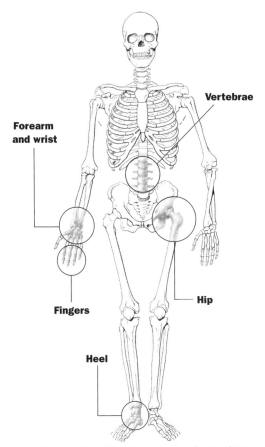

Common locations for bone density testing.

by a gradual loss of calcium and other minerals from bones, making them thinner, weaker and more prone to break.

While osteoarthritis causes stiffness and pain, osteoporosis is symptom-free at first. A bone fracture may be the first indication of a problem.

Osteoporosis is common, affecting an estimated 8 million women and 2 million men in the United States. The risk increases with age — people over age 50 are most likely to develop the disease.

Throughout your life, your bones are continuously changing. Old or worn-out bone is broken down and new bone is made. By the time most people reach their mid-30s, they begin to gradually lose bone strength as more bone is lost than is replaced.

Osteoporosis occurs when enough bone is lost that portions of your skeleton become more porous and brittle.

Your risk of developing osteoporosis depends in part on how much bone mass, or total amount of bone tissue, you developed during young adulthood and how rapidly you lose it later. Low bone mass and poor bone quality (low density) set the stage for osteoporosis. Slender, small-framed women are particularly at risk.

The sudden drop in estrogen at menopause accelerates bone loss. Not getting enough calcium and vitamin D can also speed the process. Certain medications and diseases can cause osteoporosis. For example, prolonged use of corticosteroids can lead to osteoporosis.

Who should be tested for osteoporosis?

Ideally, adults considered at risk of osteoporosis will have their bone density tested. Early testing gives them more time to start preventive measures and allow the measures to work. It's also the first and best step toward receiving a diagnosis and being treated. Remember: If the development of osteoporosis can be slowed, then prevention is your goal.

It's recommended that the following individuals have a bone density test:

- All adult women before age 65.
- Anyone over 40 who has broken a bone and is willing to undergo treatment for osteoporosis.
- All women, men and children who are at high risk of osteoporosis. Being at high risk is generally considered as having two or more risk factors.
- All women, men and children who are taking or will soon take corticosteroid drugs.
- All young adults who for any reason have a low estrogen or testosterone level.
- All adults who have a medical condition known to lower bone mass and increase the risk of fractures.

If you're a woman, consider being tested before you reach menopause, even if you have no risk factors. Menopause gener-

Signs and symptoms. Osteoporosis is a silent disease. Bone loss occurs over many years, with no symptoms. Pain associated with osteoporosis is caused by fractures of the vertebrae, hips, wrists and other bones. A compression fracture of the spine causes vertebrae to collapse and may lead to a loss of height and a stooped posture.

Diagnosis. If you're over 40 and you break a bone, you'll likely undergo diagnostic testing for osteoporosis. The primary diagnostic tools are the bone density test and a complete physical exam. Diagnostic tests are done to:

- Confirm that you have osteoporosis
- Determine the severity of your low bone density
- Establish your baseline bone density values

ally occurs around age 50. An earlier test is advisable if you're at high risk of osteoporosis or if you've broken a bone or are losing height.

Any postmenopausal woman who breaks a bone should be tested because osteoporosis will be a primary suspect for causing the fracture. If osteoporosis is the cause, the test can determine how severely you have the condition.

Bone density testing is usually not a one-time thing. Even if your bone density is normal at the initial test, plan to be retested in about five years. Bone density tests taken at intervals over several years can reveal the rate at which you may be losing bone. The rate of bone loss is a potent predictor of your fracture risk.

The frequency of retesting depends on your age and the factors that put you at risk. One to two years is the minimum amount of time for bone affected by osteoporosis to show a noticeable increase or decrease in density. If you're taking medicine to treat osteoporosis, you may benefit from an annual bone density test during the first couple of years of treatment until it's clear your bone mass is stable. Thereafter, the tests can be less frequent. If you're taking corticosteroids, it's recommended that you be tested once a year.

A bone density test is about as close as your doctor may come to foretelling the future of your bone health. By looking at the test results, he or she can tell if you have osteoporosis and give you a strong indication of your susceptibility to fracture.

Bone density tests are generally simple, fast and painless. They use special X-rays or ultrasound technology to measure how many grams of calcium and other bone minerals — collectively known as bone mineral content — are packed into a square centimeter of bone. A gram is about $\frac{1}{28th}$ of an ounce. A centimeter is about a half inch. The terms *bone mineral content* and *bone density* are often used interchangeably. The higher your mineral content, the denser your bones. The denser your bones, the stronger they are and the less likely they are to break.

Bone density tests are usually done on bones that are likely to break because of osteoporosis. These sites include the lumbar vertebrae, which are in the lower region of your spine, the narrow neck of your femur bone adjoining the hip, and the bones of your wrist or forearm (see image of skeleton on page 35).

Treatment. It's important to be aware of your risk factors. To keep your bones healthy, it's essential to get enough calcium and vitamin D. Regular exercise, especially weight-bearing exercise, also helps preserve bone strength. Depending on the results of your bone density test results, therapy to prevent further bone loss may be recommended. Several different medications may be used to prevent and treat osteoporosis. These include

- Bisphosphonates such as alendronate (Fosamax)
- Calcitonin (Calcimar, Miacalcin)
- Estrogen
- Selective estrogen receptor modulators (SERMs) such as raloxifene (Evista)
- Teriparatide (Forteo)

Chapter 3

Rheumatoid arthritis in adults and children

Rheumatoid arthritis is an inflammatory condition that can cause painful aching and swelling in your joints and leave you feeling tired and unwell. While the exact cause isn't known, the disease appears related to an abnormal response by the body's immune system.

Inflammation is the body's normal response to a foreign "invasion" such as an infection by bacteria or a virus. When the immune system identifies a threat, it activates special cells, proteins and powerful chemicals to destroy the invader. These battles result in the cardinal signs of inflammation — fever, redness, swelling, warmth and pain.

In rheumatoid arthritis and other forms of inflammatory arthritis, something goes awry with the normal immune system response. The immune system mistakenly views your own body cells as the foreign invader. The immune system cells attack your own tissues, causing inflammation. Uncontrolled, ongoing inflammation may result in damage to tissues, joints or organs.

Diseases in which the immune system attacks your own body are known as autoimmune disorders. Research shows that some people may be genetically predisposed to develop these diseases. Find out more about other forms of inflammatory arthritis in Chapter 4.

Understanding rheumatoid arthritis

About 2.1 million Americans have rheumatoid arthritis. Interestingly, some recent studies have indicated that the overall number of new cases is declining. Scientists are investigating why this is happening. Rheumatoid arthritis is two to three times more common in women than in men. It generally begins in middle age and occurs more frequently in older people. But the disease can also affect children and young adults.

In rheumatoid arthritis the inflammatory and immune reactions cause the joints to swell, ache and throb. Pain, swelling and stiffness can make even the simplest activities, such as opening a jar or taking a walk, difficult to manage. If the inflammation continues over a longer period, the joint structures suffer damage, and deformity may result.

The principal area of immune system attack in rheumatoid arthritis is the synovial membrane that lines the joints. White blood cells — whose job is to attack unwanted invaders — move from your bloodstream into your synovial membrane. The blood cells release potent chemicals that cause the membrane to become inflamed.

As the inflammation continues, more immune cells enter the synovial tissues. These cells, along with the proteins and other substances they release, cause a thickening of the normally thin membrane. The joints become painful, tender and swollen. If the inflammation persists, the inflamed synovium appears to invade and destroy cartilage, bone and soft tissues in the joint. Ligaments, muscle and bone weaken.

This weakening may lead to looseness in the joint and eventual destruction. As a result, the involved joints may gradually lose their alignment and shape. Researchers believe that rheumatoid arthritis begins to damage bones during the first year or two, which makes early diagnosis and treatment critical.

In contrast to osteoarthritis, which affects only your bones and muscles, rheumatoid arthritis can target your whole body, including parts you might not expect to be involved, such as your heart, blood vessels, lungs and eyes. However, the disease most commonly affects your joints.

Joint changes in rheumatiod arthritis

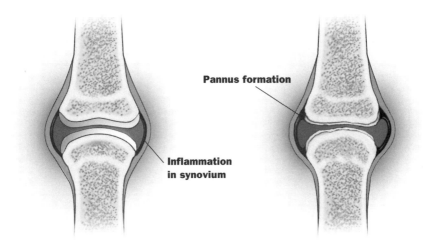

Pannus formation

Inflammation in synovium

A. Inflammation begins in the synovium. The synovium is invaded by inflammatory cells and becomes thickened. Excess synovial fluid forms. The joint becomes swollen and warm.

B. The synovium continues to proliferate. An inflammatory exudate (called pannus) forms and extends over the margins of the joint surfaces.

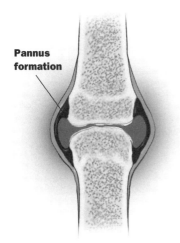

Pannus formation

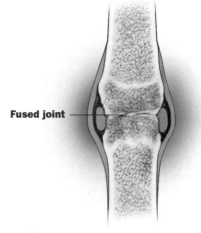

Fused joint

C. Cells in the pannus release enzymes that destroy the cartilage, bone and soft tissues of the joint. The space between the bones of the joint narrow as the cartilage is lost.

D. Tendons and the joint capsule may become inflamed, then shorten as it becomes too painful to move the joint. This results in fusion of the bones of the joint.

Having rheumatoid arthritis increases your risk of developing the bone-thinning disease osteoporosis, especially if you take corticosteroid medications. Some research suggests that people with rheumatoid arthritis also have an increased risk of infections, heart disease and certain types of cancer, such as lymphomas.

Differences between osteoarthritis and rheumatoid arthritis

Osteoarthritis	Rheumatoid Arthritis
Affects 21 million U.S. adults	Affects 2.1 million U.S. adults
Usually begins after age 40 and develops slowly	Usually begins between ages 25 and 50 and may develop suddenly, within weeks or months
Affects a few joints and may occur on one or both sides of the body	Usually affects many joints, primarily the small joints on both sides of the body
Typically affects only certain joints, most commonly those of the hips, hands, knees and lower back	Affects many joints, especially small joints of the hands and feet, and the wrists, elbows and shoulders
Usually causes minimal redness, warmth and swelling of the joints. Joints may be hard and bony. Morning stiffness is common but brief (less than 20 minutes).	Causes redness, warmth and swelling. Morning stiffness is prolonged, often lasting for hours.
Can cause Heberden's nodes, bony growths in the end joints of the fingers	Doesn't cause Heberden's nodes
Doesn't cause an overall feeling of sickness and fatigue	Often causes a general feeling of sickness and fatigue and may lead to weight loss
Blood tests are negative for rheumatoid factor; sed rate, CRP and CCP are normal (see pages 46-47)	Blood tests are often positive for rheumatoid factor; sed rate, CRP and CCP may be elevated (see pages 46-47)

What causes rheumatoid arthritis?

Although scientists have searched for decades to discover the triggering events that cause the immune response to turn against itself in rheumatoid arthritis, they still don't know exactly why this happens.

While rheumatoid arthritis itself is not inherited, certain genes that create an increased susceptibility to the disease are. People with these genes won't necessarily get rheumatoid arthritis, but they may have more of a tendency to do so. The severity of their disease may also depend on the genes inherited. At the same time, some people who don't have the genes do develop rheumatoid arthritis.

Many researchers suspect that something in the environment, such as an infectious agent, triggers the disease process in a person whose genetic makeup makes them susceptible to rheumatoid arthritis. Despite extensive efforts to identify a specific agent, such as a virus or type of bacteria, none has yet been identified.

Because women are much more likely to get rheumatoid arthritis, researchers believe that reproductive hormones such as estrogen may play a role in the disease. However, understanding of the role of hormones in the development of arthritis is limited.

Smoking increases the risk of getting rheumatoid arthritis, and cigarette smokers may have more serious forms of the disease.

Signs and symptoms

Rheumatoid arthritis affects people who have it in many different ways. One common pattern is to have periods of worsening signs and symptoms, called flares or flare-ups, and times when you feel better, called remissions. Some people have a severe form of the disease that's active most of the time and lasts for many years. For a few people, signs and symptoms last only a few months to a couple of years and then go away.

The signs and symptoms of rheumatoid arthritis vary in severity and may be constant or come and go. They include:

- Pain and swelling in your joints, especially the smaller joints of your hands and feet

- Generalized aching or stiffness of the joints and muscles, especially in the morning or after periods of rest
- Warmth and redness in a joint
- Loss of motion in the affected joints
- Weakness in muscles attached to the affected joints
- Fatigue, which can be severe during a flare
- Low-grade fever
- General sense of not feeling well
- Weight loss
- Deformity of the joints

In contrast to the morning stiffness of osteoarthritis, which usually goes away quickly, morning stiffness in rheumatoid arthritis generally lasts more than 30 minutes. On average, a person with untreated rheumatoid arthritis is stiff for about four hours after getting up in the morning.

Rheumatoid arthritis usually causes problems in several joints at the same time. While any joint may be affected, most people first experience symptoms of inflammation in the wrists, hands and feet. As the disease progresses, your knees, shoulders, elbows, hips, jaw and neck can become involved. Usually both sides of your body are affected at the same time, such as the knuckles of both hands.

Rheumatoid arthritis often is more disabling than osteoarthritis. The affected joints are swollen, painful, tender and warm during the initial attack and flares that may follow. Swelling or deformity may limit the flexibility of some joints. But even if you have a severe form of rheumatoid arthritis, you'll probably retain flexibility in many joints.

Small lumps, called rheumatoid nodules, may form under the skin over bony areas, such as your elbows, hands, knees, toes and the back of your scalp. These nodules, usually painless, range in size from that of a pea to that of a walnut.

Many people with rheumatoid arthritis develop anemia, a decrease in the number of red blood cells. Less commonly, dry eyes and dry mouth may occur. Very rarely, people with rheumatoid arthritis have inflammation of the blood vessels (vasculitis), which can cause red dots to appear on the skin. Other rare effects are inflammation of the lining of the lungs (pleurisy) or of the lining

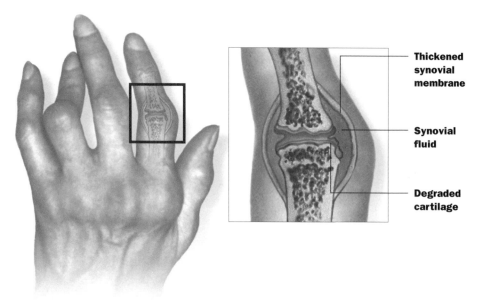

Thickened
synovial
membrane

Synovial
fluid

Degraded
cartilage

Rheumatoid arthritis often leads to deformity in fingers. During flares, your hand may be painful and weak.

surrounding the heart (pericarditis). Many people with rheumatoid arthritis also experience some degree of depression and anxiety.

Diagnosing rheumatoid arthritis

Even an experienced rheumatologist may find it difficult to determine if a person has rheumatoid arthritis or another disease that causes similar signs and symptoms. It's challenging to diagnose the disease in its early stages, especially in older people. No single test can confirm the diagnosis, and signs and symptoms vary from one person to another.

Doctors use a variety of tools to diagnose rheumatoid arthritis and rule out other conditions. Your medical history — your description of signs and symptoms and when and how they began — is an important starting point. For example, your doctor may want to know if you have morning stiffness and how long it lasts. (See "Questions your doctor may ask," page 24.) You may be given a questionnaire to fill out about your signs and symptoms.

The physical examination also yields much of the information needed to make a diagnosis. Your doctor may examine your joints, skin, reflexes and muscle strength, looking for common features of rheumatoid arthritis, such as joint swelling and tenderness and limited motion or misalignment in joints. He or she may evaluate your grip strength, walking time and other functions.

Blood tests. If you have signs and symptoms of rheumatoid arthritis, your doctor will likely order some laboratory tests. Several different types of blood tests can provide useful clues. While no test offers proof positive that you have rheumatoid arthritis, the following tests, along with the physical exam, usually provide enough information for your doctor to establish a diagnosis.

Complete blood count. Doctors often measure levels, or counts, of different types of blood cells to assess a variety of symptoms. For example, anemia (low red blood cell count) often is associated with rheumatoid arthritis and systemic lupus erythematosus. The white blood cell count is usually normal in people with rheumatoid arthritis.

Erythrocyte sedimentation rate. Sometimes referred to as "sed rate," this test determines the rate at which your red blood cells (erythrocytes) fall to the bottom of a tall, thin tube. Cells that settle faster than normal indicate the presence of inflammation, which is typical of active rheumatoid arthritis. If you have osteoarthritis, your sedimentation rate tends to be normal.

This test is easy and inexpensive. But it may be less useful for older people, since everyone's sedimentation rate increases with age, making it harder to determine a "normal" level.

C-reactive protein. C-reactive protein is made by the liver. In inflammatory illnesses, the liver quickly manufactures dramatically increased amounts of this protein, which are released into the blood. A C-reactive protein (CRP) test measures the level of this protein in your blood. In people with rheumatoid arthritis, the CRP level is typically elevated.

The CRP test is highly sensitive and generally measures small degrees of inflammation in active rheumatoid arthritis better than the sed rate. But sometimes, even during active inflammation, the CRP isn't high. Researchers don't know the reason for this.

The erythrocyte sedimentation rate and CRP tests are often used to help monitor the degree of inflammation at any given point.

Rheumatoid factor. This test identifies an antibody in your blood called rheumatoid factor. Antibodies are proteins made by cells of the immune system that normally attach to foreign substances when they enter the body. The body is then able to deactivate these substances, or germs, and eliminate them from the body. Rheumatoid factor is a type of autoantibody, which targets your body's own proteins rather than those of an outside agent.

Most people with rheumatoid arthritis have this abnormal antibody, which typically isn't present in people with osteoarthritis. Rheumatoid factor appears to be a marker of the disease and not a cause of arthritis symptoms. Rheumatoid factor is also present in some people with other diseases, so it isn't specific to rheumatoid arthritis. This test can help diagnose rheumatoid arthritis and monitor inflammation.

Cyclic citrullinated peptide (CCP) antibody. The CCP test identifies citrulline antibodies (also known as citrulline-containing peptides) in the blood. Like rheumatoid factor, citrulline antibodies are autoantibodies — proteins produced by the immune system in response to a perceived threat from one's own body, in this case from an amino acid (protein component) called citrulline.

This test can be useful in diagnosing rheumatoid arthritis early in the disease, since CCP antibodies are in the blood of half or more people with early rheumatoid arthritis. Many people who test negative for rheumatoid factor have an elevated CCP. Eventually, most people with rheumatoid arthritis have CCP antibodies.

Imaging tests

In addition to blood tests, your doctor may order X-ray examinations to look for damage to affected joints. A sequence of X-rays obtained over time can show the progression of rheumatoid arthritis. As the disease progresses, many people develop erosions (small holes) near the ends of the bones in joints and narrowing of the space around the joint because of cartilage loss.

Because it often takes several months of active inflammation before damage appears on an X-ray, your doctor may not order

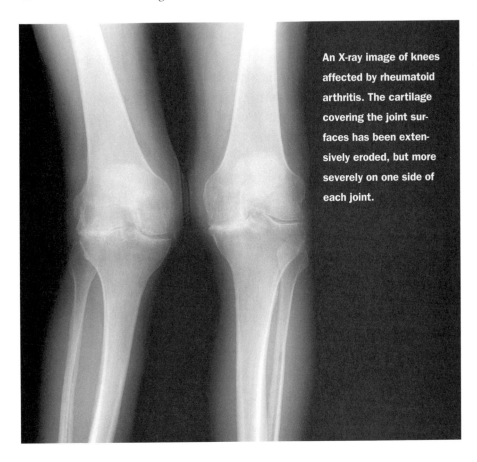

An X-ray image of knees affected by rheumatoid arthritis. The cartilage covering the joint surfaces has been extensively eroded, but more severely on one side of each joint.

X-rays if your symptoms have just developed. An MRI (magnetic resonance imaging) scan can detect early inflammation and cartilage damage that would not be seen on an X-ray. MRI is useful in detecting early rheumatoid arthritis.

Treatment
Thanks to better treatments and self-care techniques, most people with rheumatoid arthritis can avoid the most severe, disabling consequences of the disease. Newer drugs are more effective and have fewer side effects than traditional medications. Doctors often use these drugs in combination early in the disease to control inflammation and prevent joint damage.

Treatment varies from one person to another and at different times during the course of the disease. The goals of treatment are to relieve pain, reduce inflammation, slow or stop joint damage, and improve your well-being and ability to carry out your normal activities. A variety of treatment approaches may be used, including exercise programs and physical therapy, joint protection and self-care methods. Most people will use one or more medications. In some cases, surgical procedures may be necessary.

You can learn more about treatments for rheumatoid arthritis in later chapters in this book, which deal with self-care techniques, medications, alternative treatments, surgery and new therapies on the horizon.

A chronic disease

When you're first diagnosed, it's impossible to predict how severe your rheumatoid arthritis may eventually be. It may be mild or progressive. For most people, the disease becomes chronic, although it tends to vary in severity at different times. Flares alternate with periods of relative remission. Early diagnosis and treatment may help you avoid persistent pain and permanent joint damage.

If you have fairly continuous symptoms for four or five years, your condition is more likely to pose a long-standing challenge. Your doctor will likely monitor the disease with periodic examination of your joints and various tests. After 10 to 20 years, the symptoms of inflammation, especially joint swelling, may stabilize, but joint deformities and some pain may remain.

There's no known cure for rheumatoid arthritis, but with proper treatment, exercise, joint protection and changes in lifestyle, most people live long, productive lives after their arthritis develops.

Juvenile rheumatoid arthritis

Juvenile rheumatoid arthritis (JRA), also called juvenile idiopathic arthritis (JIA), refers to chronic conditions that cause joint inflammation in children age 16 or younger. The word *idiopathic* means the cause is unknown — the exact causes of JRA remain unclear.

Like adult rheumatoid arthritis, juvenile arthritis is an autoimmune disorder that involves both genetic and environmental factors.

Nearly 300,000 children in the United States have some form of juvenile arthritis. It's one of the most common chronic childhood illnesses. Only a small number of children with arthritis still continue to have it as adults.

JRA is divided into several subtypes based on the features of the disease. The major categories include:

- **Pauciarticular JRA.** Also known as oligoarthritis, this is the most common form of the disease, affecting about half of children with arthritis. Pauciarthritis affects four or fewer joints — typically the larger joints such as the knees and ankles. Often only one knee is affected. Girls are more likely to have this form of arthritis than are boys.

  Most commonly, pauciarthritis occurs in children before the age of 4. The disease may subside over time. But older children with pauciarthritis often develop an extended disease that involves multiple joints and lasts into adulthood.

- **Polyarticular JRA.** About one-third of children with JRA have this type, called polyarticular JRA. *Poly* means "many," and this form of arthritis affects five or more joints — typically small joints, such as those in the hands and feet. It often affects the same joint on both sides of the body. Poly-arthritis can begin at any age and affects girls more often than boys.

- **Systemic onset JRA.** Ten percent to 20 percent of children with JRA have this subtype, also known as systemic-onset JRA, or Still's disease. Systemic onset arthritis affects many areas of the body, including joints and internal organs. The disease often begins with a fever and rash that come and go. Joint symptoms may not show up until months or even years after the onset of fevers.

- **Other types of juvenile arthritis.** Enthesitis-related arthritis (ERA) includes a group of diseases that involve the joints of the back and pelvis. Enthesitis refers to inflammation of the enthesis, the place where ligaments and tendons attach to bone. These diseases, including juvenile ankylosing spondylitis, are most common in boys over age 8 and involve a strong genetic component.

Another type of juvenile arthritis is psoriatic arthritis. Children with this form have both arthritis and psoriasis, a skin disease. Psoriatic arthritis and ERA are the least common forms of JRA.

Signs and symptoms

Signs and symptoms of JRA vary from one child to another. They can fluctuate from day to day and even throughout the same day. They may include:

- **Joint swelling, with pain and stiffness.** This may be more pronounced in the morning or after a nap. Children may not complain of joint pain. Rather, you might notice them limping. Or they may be less active than usual or be reluctant to use an arm or leg. Parents may notice a change or difficulty in the way a child crawls, walks, runs, jumps, colors, writes, ties shoes, eats, or holds a cup or spoon.
- **Fever and rash.** These are characteristic signs of systemic arthritis. The fever and rash may appear and disappear quickly. Children with systemic arthritis may also have swollen lymph nodes.
- **Eye inflammation.** This tends to occur mostly in children with pauciarthritis. Signs and symptoms of eye inflammation can include red eyes, eye pain and increased pain when looking at light. In about half of children with pauciarticular JRA who have eye inflammation, pain may not be present. Routine eye examinations are recommended because eye inflammation may result in blindness.

Like other forms of arthritis, JRA includes times when symptoms are present (flares) and times when symptoms disappear (remissions).

Diagnosis

The diagnosis of JRA is based on a medical history and physical exam. Some blood tests that can help pinpoint the diagnosis include:

- **Erythrocyte sedimentation (sed) rate.** As with rheumatoid arthritis, an elevated sed rate can indicate inflammation. This test may be used to rule out other conditions and determine the degree of inflammation.
- **Anti-nuclear antibodies.** These are immune system proteins commonly produced in people with certain autoimmune diseases, including arthritis. Anti-nuclear antibodies are present in about 40 percent of children with juvenile arthritis.

In addition to these lab tests, X-rays may be taken to exclude other conditions, such as fractures, tumors, infection and birth defects. X-rays may also be used from time to time after the diagnosis to monitor bone development and possible joint damage.

The doctor may also remove some fluid from the child's swollen joint. This can relieve pain and can help the doctor identify the cause of the arthritis.

Treatment

Treatment for JRA depends on the child's type of arthritis and his or her symptoms. For all children, treatment focuses on maintaining a normal level of physical and social activity. To accomplish this, doctors may use a combination of strategies to relieve pain and swelling, maintain full movement and strength, and prevent complications. A treatment program may include medications, exercise, eye care, dental care and good nutrition.

Medications are used to relieve pain and swelling and limit progression of the disease. Initial treatment often includes nonsteroidal anti-inflammatory drugs (NSAIDs) and corticosteroids. Use of disease-modifying antirheumatic drugs (DMARDs) and biologic agents can also help many children with JRA. These medications are discussed in detail in Chapter 5, starting on page 102.

Parents can help children with JRA by encouraging a positive outlook and physical activity. Family members can also help children cope with the emotional aspects of having a chronic disease.

Chapter 4

Other inflammatory arthritic and connective tissue disorders

In addition to osteoarthritis and rheumatoid arthritis, more than 100 other conditions are considered forms of arthritis. Many are uncommon. However, doctors are regularly recognizing new arthritic syndromes and new subtypes of old ones. Some forms are mild and resolve quickly with treatment. Others involve the body in a widespread manner, affecting multiple organs and blood vessels.

The signs and symptoms of different forms of arthritis vary, even among people with the same type. But symptoms of different forms of arthritis often overlap, which can make diagnosing particular forms challenging.

As with rheumatoid arthritis, genetic factors play a role in other forms of arthritis. Some genes have been identified that are associated with particular types of arthritis. Even if you inherit a tendency to develop arthritis, however, other factors are involved in triggering the disease. Some of the more common forms of arthritis are discussed below.

Gout

Gout is a painful form of arthritis that's been recognized since ancient times. It causes sudden, severe attacks of pain, tenderness,

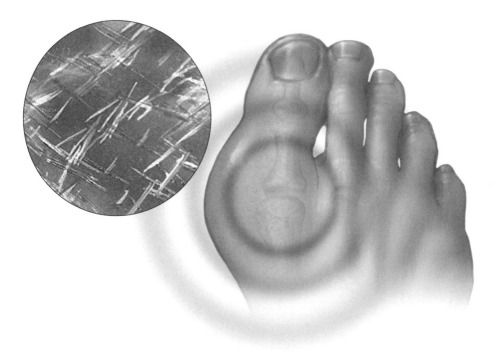

Gout occurs when an you have an excessive amount of uric acid in your system. Tiny crystals form in the joints, commonly in your feet, and can cause intense pain, inflammation and redness.

redness, warmth and swelling in some joints. It usually affects one joint at a time — typically the large joint of the big toe. But it also can occur in your feet, ankles, knees, hands and wrists.

Gout affects about 2.2 million Americans, most often men between ages 40 and 50. Although men are more likely than women to get gout, women become more susceptible to it after menopause.

Gout is caused by an excessive level of uric acid — a normal waste product — in your blood. Normally, uric acid dissolves in your blood, is filtered by your kidneys and is excreted in your urine. But sometimes the body produces too much uric acid, or, more commonly, the kidneys are unable to remove it adequately. When uric acid builds up, it can form microscopic crystals in and around the joints. These crystals set off an intense inflammatory reaction.

Signs and symptoms. Gout attacks usually come on suddenly, often at night. You may go to bed feeling fine, but then wake up in the middle of the night with your big toe feeling like it's on fire, with severe pain and swelling. The affected joint may be red or purple, hot and extremely tender.

The pain typically lasts five to 10 days, then disappears completely. You may have a period of no symptoms at all, followed by other acute episodes. An episode of gout can be triggered by drinking too much alcohol, eating too much of certain foods, surgery, severe illness or a joint injury.

If gout isn't treated, after a number of years it may lead to persistent swelling, stiffness and pain in one or more joints. Uric acid crystals may also build up into large deposits called tophi (TOE-fye), which look like lumps beneath the skin around the joints.

Diagnosis. Gout is diagnosed by identifying crystals in fluid that's drawn (aspirated) from an inflamed joint.

Treatment. NSAIDs can help relieve the pain and inflammation of a gout attack. Once the acute attack is under control, your doctor may prescribe a medication to reduce the risk of future episodes. Preventive medications include allopurinol (Zyloprim, Aloprim) and probenecid. They help keep uric acid levels within a normal range. You may also need to watch your diet by avoiding too much animal protein, limiting alcohol and drinking plenty of water.

Pseudogout

In pseudogout (SOO-doe-gout), also known as calcium pyrophosphate deposition disease (CPPD), calcium salt crystals build up in the joint cartilage. When these crystals are released into the joint cavity, they set off an episode of joint pain and swelling. Although the symptoms are similar to those of gout, pseudogout is caused by a different type of crystal. The two forms of arthritis also occur in different joints. Gout most often affects the big toe, while in pseudogout, the affected joint is more likely to be your knee, wrist or ankle.

Anyone can get pseudogout, but it occurs most often in adults in their 60s or older. The disease can occur with no obvious cause or during recovery from acute illness or surgery. Genetic factors may play a role. Joint injury, osteoarthritis, underactive thyroid or excess storage of iron can also contribute.

Signs and symptoms. Severe attacks of pseudogout can occur abruptly, causing pain, swelling and warmth in the affected joint. Usually just a single joint is involved, most commonly the knee or wrist.

Diagnosis. Like gout, pseudogout can be diagnosed by examining fluid from an affected joint to see whether calcium crystals are present. An X-ray often shows calcified cartilage, known as chondrocalcinosis.

Treatment. NSAIDs such as indomethacin (Indocin) and naproxen (Aleve, Naprosyn) can help relieve pain and inflammation. Another option, especially for a large joint such as the knee, may be an injection of a corticosteroid drug. Your doctor may remove the calcium crystals from your joint by suctioning out the fluid. To prevent further attacks, low doses of colchicine (available only as a generic) or NSAIDs may be effective.

Pseudogout and gout — What's the difference?

Disease	Cause	Signs and symptoms	Who does it affect?	Treatment
Pseudogout	Deposits of calcium pyrophosphate dihydrate crystals in joints	Pain and swelling, usually in large joints such as the knee	Typically older adults	NSAIDs, steroids, colchicine
Gout	Deposits of uric acid crystals in joints	Pain and swelling, usually in metatarsal joint of big toe	Typically older men	NSAIDs, colchicine, allopurinol (Aloprim, Zyloprim) and probenecid

Spondyloarthropathy

The word *spondyloarthropathy* (spon-duh-lo-ahr-THROP-uh-thee) refers to a group of autoimmune disorders that cause inflammation in the sacroiliac joints of the lower spine, the sites where tendons attach to bones in the spine (entheses), and joints of the lower extremities and toes. Often, the arthritis is asymmetrical, affecting only one side of the body. Diseases in this group include ankylosing spondylitis, reactive arthritis, psoriatic arthritis and arthritis associated with inflammatory bowel disease. People who don't have the distinctive signs and symptoms of one of these four conditions are classified as having "undifferentiated" spondyloarthropathy.

This group of conditions is thought to affect almost 2 percent of the population. Like the other forms of arthritis, spondyloarthropathies appear to stem from a combination of genetic and environmental factors. Many people with spondyloarthropathy have the HLA-B27 gene.

Signs and symptoms. People with spondyloarthropathy can experience inflamed, painful joints in the knees, ankles and feet, as well as low back and neck pain. Often the back pain starts before age 40 and gradually gets worse. You may have prolonged morning stiffness that improves with activity.

People with this form of arthritis may also have a painful eye inflammation and bowel problems.

Diagnosis. Your doctor will base the diagnosis on your symptoms and physical examination. X-rays, CT scans and MRI images can also help with the diagnosis. For example, an X-ray of your foot may show changes typical of this condition.

Blood tests can help rule out other forms of arthritis. You may also be tested for the HLA-B27 gene.

Treatment. Physical therapy and exercise, including stretching and range-of-motion exercises, can help people with spondyloarthropathy maintain flexibility in joints and good posture. Several types of medications may be used to control inflammation. These include NSAIDs, corticosteroids, DMARDs and biologic agents, all of which are discussed in depth in Chapter 5.

Ankylosing spondylitis

Ankylosing spondylitis (ang-kuh-LOE-sing spon-duh-LI-tis) primarily causes inflammation between the vertebrae of your spine and in the joints between your spine and pelvis (sacroiliac joints). It may also cause inflammation in sites where your tendons and ligaments attach to bones (entheses), the joints between your ribs and spine, the joints of your hips, shoulders, knees and feet, and your eyes, heart and lungs.

Ankylosing spondylitis (AS) is more common in men than in women and usually begins between the ages of 20 to 40. It affects about 300,000 people in the United States.

The majority of people with ankylosing spondylitis have a gene called HLA-B27. Having this gene doesn't mean that you'll get the disease — only about 2 percent of people who have the gene develop AS — but it may make you more susceptible. Other genes also likely play a role. About 15 percent to 20 percent of people with AS have a family history of the disease.

Signs and symptoms. Early signs and symptoms often include pain and stiffness in your lower back and hips, or a dull aching deep in your buttocks. The pain may come and go at first and is often worse in the morning, at night and after periods of inactivity. Loss of flexibility in the lower spine is an early sign of AS. Over time, pain and stiffness may progress up your spine and to other joints, such as those in your hips, shoulders, knees and feet.

AS is a chronic condition. As inflammation persists, new bone forms as part of the healing process. The vertebrae may begin to grow or fuse together, forming vertical bony outgrowths and becoming stiff and inflexible. Fusion can also stiffen your rib cage, restricting lung capacity and function. In advanced stages, signs and symptoms may include chronic stooping, a stiff, inflexible spine, fatigue, loss of appetite, weight loss, eye inflammation (iritis) and bowel inflammation.

Many people with AS have mild disease that involves only a small area, while others have a more severe case that leads to physical deformities and other complications.

Diagnosis. Early diagnosis of AS can be difficult if your symptoms are mild, since you may attribute them to more common back problems. If your doctor suspects AS based on your medical history and signs and symptoms, he or she may order X-rays to check for changes in your joints and bones, though the characteristic effects of the disease aren't evident early on. Blood tests to check for an elevated sed rate (see page 46) and for the presence of the HLA-B27 gene can help confirm the diagnosis.

Treatment. Effective treatment can decrease your pain and may help prevent complications and physical deformities. Stretching and breathing exercises, proper posture and physical therapy are key aspects of treatment. Nonsteroidal anti-inflammatory drugs (see page 83) can relieve pain and inflammation, and medications that block tumor necrosis factor (TNF) (see page 114) are very effective in improving signs and symptoms and quality of life. Many people with ankylosing spondylitis can lead normal, active lives.

Reactive arthritis

Reactive arthritis is an inflammatory condition that occurs as a reaction to an infection elsewhere in your body. Many different types of infectious organisms can trigger arthritis. What's considered the classic form of reactive arthritis is triggered by a bacterial infection in the intestines or the urogenital area. The intestinal form is caused by food-borne infections from salmonella, campylobacter, shigella or yersinia. Chlamydia and gonorrhea, two sexually transmitted infections, can cause the genital form of reactive arthritis.

Reactive arthritis was formerly known as Reiter's syndrome. It's another in the group of disorders known as the spondyloarthropathies, which also includes ankylosing spondylitis (page 58) and psoriatic arthritis (see page 60). These diseases can cause inflammation throughout the body, especially in the spine, legs and arms.

Not everyone who is exposed to a bacterial infection gets arthritis. Reactive arthritis is thought to be triggered in people who are genetically predisposed to it — they have inherited a gene or genes that make them more likely to get arthritis. More than three-fourths of people with reactive arthritis have a gene called HLA-B27. But having this gene doesn't necessarily mean you'll get reactive arthritis if you're exposed to an infection. Overall, men between the ages of 20 and 40 are most likely to develop reactive arthritis.

Signs and symptoms. Reactive arthritis typically involves pain and swelling in the knees, ankles, feet and hips. Other joints, such as the wrists and fingers, are affected less often. Inflammation of the tendons (tendinitis) or at places where tendons attach to bones (enthesitis) is common. This often results in heel pain or pain at the back of the ankle. About half of people with reactive arthritis have pain in the lower back and buttocks.

Although joint symptoms are a defining feature of reactive arthritis, the condition can also cause inflammation in your eyes, skin and the tube that carries urine from your bladder (urethra). This can lead to skin rashes, eye conditions, increased urinary frequency and a burning sensation during urination.

The signs and symptoms generally start days to weeks after exposure to a triggering infection. Signs and symptoms may come and go over a period of several weeks or months. In some people, they subside within a few days, and most people recover within a year. But up to half of people redevelop signs and symptoms after their initial condition disappears.

Diagnosis. Reactive arthritis can go undetected for some time because signs and symptoms may be mild. Your doctor may perform tests to see if you have any of the infections that are often associated with reactive arthritis. Blood tests, such as those for sed rate, rheumatoid factor and antinuclear antibodies, can help determine what type of arthritis you have. You may undergo a blood test to see if you carry the HLA-B27 gene.

Treatment. Treatment may involve antibiotics to eliminate the bacterial infection that triggered reactive arthritis. Your doctor may prescribe NSAIDs (page 83) and corticosteroid medications (page 94) to relieve joint pain and inflammation. Drugs that inhibit a protein called tumor necrosis factor (page 113) may also be used to treat reactive arthritis.

Psoriatic arthritis

Among the approximately 6 million Americans who have the skin disease psoriasis, between 20 percent and 30 percent develop a chronic, inflammatory arthritis, known as psoriatic (sor-ee-AT-ik) arthritis. In addition to the inflamed, scaly skin that's typical of psoriasis, people with psoriatic arthritis have swollen, painful joints — especially in their fingers and toes — and pitted, discolored nails. They may also develop inflammatory eye conditions such as conjunctivitis.

Psoriatic arthritis affects men and women equally. Most people with the condition have psoriasis long before they develop arthritic symptoms. Psoriasis typically develops in adults in their 20s or 30s, while psoriatic arthritis may show up 20 years later. Children can also get psoriatic arthritis, usually between ages 9 and 12.

Both psoriasis and the arthritis associated with it are autoimmune conditions. Most people with psoriatic arthritis have a close relative with the disease, and researchers have discovered certain gene mutations that appear to be associated with it. Among people with a genetic predisposition to develop psoriatic arthritis, something in the environment, such as a viral or bacterial infection or physical trauma, may trigger the disease.

Signs and symptoms. Psoriasis is a skin condition marked by a buildup of rough, dry, dead skin cells that form thick scales. These patches, or plaques, of thick, red skin often appear on your elbows, knees, scalp or the lower part of your spine. Your fingernails may become pitted and discolored and separate from the nail beds.

Arthritic symptoms include pain, redness, swelling and reduced motion in your joints, especially the small joints at the ends of your fingers and toes. The joints in your spine and your sacroiliac joints (which connect your pelvis and sacrum, the triangular bone at the end of the spine) may also be affected. Morning stiffness lasting more than 30 minutes is common, as is stiffness following periods of inactivity.

Different types of psoriatic arthritis cause varying symptoms. For example, in a mild type called asymmetric arthritis, inflammation of the tendons in your fingers and toes can cause them to swell up like small sausages. In a rare form called spondylitis, inflammation in the spine can make movement painful and difficult.

Diagnosis. To be diagnosed with psoriatic arthritis, you have to have symptoms of both psoriasis and arthritis. This diagnosis can be tricky because in adults, the skin and joint problems rarely begin at the same time.

Arthritis and inflammatory bowel disease

More than 1 million people have Crohn's disease or ulcerative colitis, the two most common forms of inflammatory bowel disease (IBD). These conditions cause chronic inflammation of the digestive tract. Up to 20 percent of people with IBD also experience arthritis, known as enteropathic arthritis.

Because people with this condition often experience pain and swelling in multiple joints, especially the knees and ankles, and stiffness in the spine, this condition is grouped as a type of spondyloarthropy.

Some researchers think that the arthritis in spondyloarthropathies may result from an immune response to intestinal bacteria in the inflamed bowel.

Your doctor may order blood tests to check your sed rate and test for rheumatoid factor to rule out rheumatoid arthritis. X-rays may show changes in the joints that develop in psoriatic arthritis but not in other arthritic conditions.

Treatment. For most people with psoriatic arthritis, the condition is a nuisance rather than a significant problem. If you have a mild form of the disease, your doctor may recommend NSAIDs such as aspirin or ibuprofen. If these medications don't control your pain and inflammation, you may be treated with DMARDs (see page 102) or biologic agents (page 113). In addition, various treatments, including oral medications, ointments and creams, and ultraviolet light or sunlight (phototherapy) are used for skin symptoms.

Sjogren's syndrome

Although mild decreases in saliva and tears can be normal with aging, if you have Sjogren's (SHOW-grins) syndrome, your tear and saliva glands become inflamed, which markedly interferes with the flow of tears and saliva. The result is a dry mouth and a sandy, gritty feeling in your eyes.

Sjogren's syndrome is an autoimmune disease that may occur by itself or along with rheumatoid arthritis, systemic lupus erythematosus, scleroderma or polymyositis. In Sjogren's syndrome, the main targets of the attack by your immune system are the mucous membranes and glands that produce moisture, primarily in your eyes and mouth. The disease may also cause vaginal dryness in women and problems in the muscles, joints, lungs, kidneys and stomach.

Sjogren's syndrome affects about 1 million to 4 million Americans. Middle-aged women are at highest risk — the disease is nine times more likely to occur in women than in men. Researchers believe that many factors, including an inherited tendency, contribute to the development of Sjogren's syndrome.

Signs and symptoms. The classic symptoms are dry mouth and dry eyes. Your eyes may feel as if foreign bodies are lodged in them, and you may have difficulty swallowing or chewing. Other signs and symptoms include:

- Dental cavities
- Fatigue
- A dry nose, throat and lungs, causing a dry cough or hoarseness
- Muscle and joint pain and joint swelling and stiffness
- Mucus-like strands in the eyes, especially in the morning
- Enlarged salivary glands behind your jaw and in front of your ears
- Skin rashes, including purple spots
- Shortness of breath
- Change in sense of taste
- Nausea, stomach pain or indigestion
- Raynaud's phenomenon (numbness, pain or color changes in your skin brought on by cold or stress)
- Vaginal dryness

Diagnosis. Your doctor may ask for a history of your symptoms and do a physical exam, including an eye exam. He or she may also order blood tests and a lip biopsy, in which a sample of lip tissue containing small salivary glands is removed for analysis. Your doctor can measure the dryness of your eyes by way of a special eye examination or with a Schirmer's tear test, in which a small piece of filter paper is placed under your lower eyelid to measure your tears. To determine if inflammation is damaging your salivary glands, you may have a special X-ray called a sialogram.

Treatment. Most people with Sjogren's syndrome can ease many symptoms with a self-care plan that includes using artificial tears, eyedrops and moisturizers, avoiding dry environments, sucking sugarless candy and drinking plenty of fluids. Your doctor can review any medications you take to make sure they aren't contributing to your symptoms.

To relieve pain and inflammation, your doctor may prescribe NSAIDs or corticosteroids. Pilocarpine (Salagen) is a prescription medication for dry eyes and dry mouth, and cevimeline (Evoxac) can relieve dry mouth symptoms. Some people whose joint pain and inflammation aren't relieved by NSAIDs may benefit from a DMARD such as hydroxychloroquine (Plaquenil) (see page 103).

Systemic lupus erythematosus

Systemic lupus erythematosus (er-uh-them-uh-TO-sus), often called simply lupus or SLE, is a chronic inflammatory disease that can affect many parts of your body, including your skin, joints, kidneys, blood cells, heart and lungs. The most common symptoms include arthritis and skin rashes. Episodes of lupus tend to come and go throughout your life, and they may make you feel tired and achy.

Nine out of 10 people with SLE are women. It's most commonly diagnosed between the ages of 15 and 45. But it can occur at any age and in either sex. The disease is more common in black American women and women of Hispanic, Asian and Native American descent.

SLE is also an autoimmune disorder. Sometimes SLE and related conditions are referred to as connective tissue diseases. Other diseases considered as connective tissue diseases include scleroderma (see page 66), polymyositis and dermatomyositis (see page 67), and vasculitis (see page 71).

Signs and symptoms. Symptoms of SLE vary from one person to another. They may be mild or severe, and you may have times when you experience no signs or symptoms.

Fatigue, often severe and prolonged, is the most common symptom among people with SLE, affecting almost everyone who has the disease. You may still feel tired even when no other symptoms are present. Arthritis symptoms are also very common and may be the earliest manifestation of the disease. You may experience joint pain, stiffness and swelling, especially in your fingers, hands, wrists and knees.

Other signs and symptoms include:
- Fever
- Weight loss
- A butterfly-shaped rash across the bridge of your nose and cheeks, or a scaly, disk-shaped rash on your face, neck or chest
- Sensitivity to sunlight
- Raynaud's phenomenon (see page 67)
- Mouth or nose ulcers (painless sores)
- Chest pain or cough
- Hair loss
- Swollen glands or swelling in your legs or around your eyes

Diagnosis. If your doctor suspects lupus based on your symptoms, the diagnosis may be confirmed by a series of blood tests. One of these is called the anti-nuclear antibody (ANA) test. Anti-nuclear antibodies are proteins produced by the immune system. They are found in the blood of nearly all people with systemic lupus erythematosus. However, a positive ANA doesn't mean you have lupus. People with other autoimmune diseases as well as some healthy individuals may test positive for ANA. Your doctor may advise testing for antibodies that are more specific to SLE, such as anti-DNA or other anti-nuclear antibodies, to confirm the diagnosis.

In addition to ordering blood tests, your doctor may evaluate how well your kidney, liver, chest and heart are functioning.

A diagnosis of lupus can seem scary, since in the past the disease was often considered fatal. But the majority of people with lupus today can expect to live a normal life span.

Treatment. Your treatment plan will depend on your symptoms and how severe they are. Most treatments aim to reduce inflammation, control joint pain and fatigue, and avoid complications. Medications used to control inflammation include NSAIDs such as aspirin, ibuprofen or naproxen, the antimalarial drug hydroxychloroquine (Plaquenil; see page 103), corticosteroids and immunosuppressants such as mycophenolate (Cellcept), cyclophosphamide (Cytoxan) and azathioprine (Imuran). These medications are discussed in Chapter 5. More aggressive therapy may be needed if your symptoms are more serious.

Scleroderma

Scleroderma (sklere-o-DER-muh) means "hard skin." The term encompasses a group of rare disorders that cause hardening and tightening of your skin and connective tissues. Like other connective tissue diseases, scleroderma is an autoimmune condition. It occurs when the body produces too much collagen, a fibrous protein that makes up the connective tissues. Deposits of collagen then accumulate in body tissues.

Scleroderma usually begins with puffy hands and feet. You may have a few dry patches of skin on the hands, arms or face that begin getting thicker and harder. Other areas of your skin may be involved later. In some cases, the disease can affect the blood vessels and internal organs.

Researchers aren't sure what causes this abnormal production of collagen. The disease is more common in women than in men and typically affects middle-aged adults.

Signs and symptoms. Signs and symptoms of scleroderma vary, depending on the form of the disease you have. Skin abnormalities, such as hardening and thickening, are a common feature. The hands and face are usually affected first, becoming puffy. Your skin may lose its elasticity and become shiny as it stretches across underlying bone. Other symptoms may include stiffness or pain in your joints, curling of your fingers, sores over joints, and digestive problems if the intestines become involved.

People with scleroderma often experience Raynaud's phenomenon. In Raynaud's phenomenon, spasms of blood vessels in your hands cause color changes in the skin in areas affected. Typically in an episode of Raynaud's phenomenon, one or more fingers become pale and look white as the spasm in the arteries prevents blood from reaching the fingers. Later the fingers become blue as the fingers develop a lack of oxygen. Finally, when the arteries open, the fingers turn red as new blood enters the area. In some instances the color changes are not as distinct. These symptoms are typically brought on by exposure to cold or stress.

Diagnosis. Early on, scleroderma can resemble rheumatoid arthritis or lupus, making diagnosis challenging. Your doctor likely will review your symptoms and medical history and check your skin for thickened and hardened areas. He or she may examine your joints and tendons to look for possible connective tissue changes.

Other tests may include blood tests and a tissue sample (biopsy) of your affected skin.

Treatment. Although there's no treatment to stop the overproduction of collagen that occurs in scleroderma, your doctor may recommend a number of treatments to control your symptoms. For skin problems, topical treatments such as moisturizers or a corticosteroid cream may be used. Other skin treatments may include light therapy, laser surgery and oral medications.

Several different types of medications, including calcium channel blockers, alpha blockers and low-dose aspirin, can help with circulation problems. To control joint pain, stiffness and inflammation, your doctor may prescribe NSAIDs and DMARDs.

Because scleroderma can take a toll on your self-esteem, a support group or counseling may be helpful.

Polymyositis and dermatomyositis

These two rare conditions are forms of myositis, a disease that causes inflammation within muscle tissues. Polymyositis (pol-e-mi-o-SI-tis) can cause inflammation and weakness of virtually all of your muscles. When a skin rash accompanies the muscle inflammation, the disorder is called dermatomyositis (*dermato* means "skin").

Adults between the ages of 30 and 60 are most likely to have these disorders. Dermatomyositis can also affect children, usually between the ages of 5 and 14. Both disorders are more common in women than in men, and among blacks than among whites.

The cause of these diseases isn't known, but they're thought to be autoimmune disorders.

Signs and symptoms. Muscle weakness is the most common symptom of both disorders. The weakness usually begins gradually and gets worse over a period of months. It typically affects both the right and left sides of your body, particularly the muscles closest to the trunk, such as those in the hips, thighs, shoulders, upper arms and neck. You may also have pain and swelling in your small joints.

Weakness can make it hard to do things like comb your hair, put on clothes, climb stairs, and get in and out of a bathtub, bed, chair or car. Weakness in the throat muscles can make swallowing difficult. Lung problems may also develop.

Dermatomyositis causes several types of rashes, including reddish patches of skin on the face, knuckles, elbows, knees or ankles. Rashes may also appear around the eyes and on the eyelids, or on the upper back and neck and along the sides of the arms.

Diagnosis. Polymyositis and dermatomyositis can be difficult to diagnose. Your doctor may need to perform a variety of tests and see you several times before pinpointing the diagnosis. A physical exam will be done to check your skin and test your muscle strength. Blood tests are used to check for elevated levels of certain muscle enzymes, which can indicate muscle damage.

Other tests that may be performed include electromyography, which measures the electrical activity in your muscles, and magnetic resonance imaging (MRI), which can show areas of muscle inflammation. Your doctor may do a biopsy of affected muscles — a small piece of muscle tissue is removed surgically for microscopic study to determine the amount and type of muscle damage.

Treatment. Treatment can improve your muscle strength and function. Treatment usually begins with a high dose of a corticosteroid medication. After the first month or so, the dosage is gradually lowered to the lowest effective dose. If a steroid medication doesn't improve symptoms, your doctor may recommend an immunosuppressant drug such as azathioprine or methotrexate (page 104).

Exercise and physical therapy are also helpful. People with dermatomyositis should protect themselves from exposure to sunlight by using sunscreen, wearing a hat and avoiding the sun during the middle of the day.

Rheumatic fever

Rheumatic fever is an inflammatory disease that can affect many parts of your body, including your joints, heart, brain and skin. Rheumatic fever begins with a streptoccocal throat infection. Scarlet fever is also caused by an infection with a certain strain of streptococcal germs.

Symptoms of rheumatic fever generally appear within five weeks after an untreated strep infection. But most cases of strep throat, even those that aren't treated, don't lead to rheumatic fever.

Anyone can get rheumatic fever, but it primarily affects children between ages 5 and 15. The disease occurs worldwide. It's occurred far less frequently in the United States since the beginning of the 20th century, but there have been some outbreaks since the late 1980s.

Sometimes rheumatic fever causes long-term or permanent damage to the heart valves. This is known as rheumatic heart disease, and it may not be discovered until years later.

Signs and symptoms. A strep infection may cause a sore throat, red, swollen tonsils, fever, headache and muscle aches. In up to a third of cases, though, the strep infection doesn't cause any symptoms. Symptoms of rheumatic fever usually begin one to six weeks later and include:
- Fever
- Fatigue
- Joint pain, most commonly involving the knees, elbows, wrists and ankles

Infectious arthritis

In addition to the bacteria that can cause reactive arthritis, other types of microorganisms can trigger arthritic symptoms. For example, joint pain is a common symptom of Lyme disease. If you're bitten by a tick carrying the Borrelia burgdorferi organism, you may get Lyme disease. As the infection spreads in the skin from the site of the bite, a red or pink oval or disk-shaped rash may appear. This is followed by fever, chills, sore throat, fatigue and nausea.

If the infection remains untreated, the organisms may spread to other areas in the body. Weeks later, stiffness, sharp pain and swelling may occur in your joints. The pain may affect one joint for a few days, then disappear and reappear in another joint. Left untreated, Lyme disease can result in chronic joint inflammation (Lyme arthritis), particularly in your knee. Other organs, such as your heart or brain, may be affected as well.

Less commonly, your joints may become directly infected by a germ entering your blood. If, for example, a boil or other infection releases staphylococcal bacteria into your blood, these bacteria can spread to a knee or some other joint. The infection causes the characteristic reaction of inflammation — swelling, redness, heat and pain. The pain is usually intense and sudden. If untreated, bacterial joint infections usually rapidly cause damage to the joint.

In addition to bacteria, several viruses, including hepatitis B and C, German measles (rubella), mumps, parvovirus B19, Epstein-Barr and HIV, can also cause arthritis symptoms. Viral arthritis tends to affect several joints on both sides of your body. Joint pain may come on suddenly and may be accompanied by a rash. This type of arthritis usually doesn't last long.

- Joint swelling, redness or warmth
- Chest pain and shortness of breath
- Areas of pink rash with clear centers
- Abdominal pain
- Pea-sized lumps under your skin, usually over bony areas
- Involuntary jerky movements of your limbs and face or more subtle movement difficulties, such as problems with handwriting
- Emotional disturbances, such as crying or restlessness

The arthritis that goes along with rheumatic fever usually affects several joints in quick succession, each for a short time. The arthritis seems to move from one joint to another.

Diagnosis. Diagnosis typically includes a physical examination of heart sounds, skin and joints and taking blood samples to test for evidence of a recent strep infection. Other blood tests may also be done, as well as an electrocardiogram (ECG) of the heart, which checks for abnormal heartbeats.

Treatment. Most people with rheumatic fever need to go to a hospital for initial treatment. You may be given penicillin or another antibiotic to kill the strep bacteria. To control fever, joint pain and inflammation, your doctor may prescribe aspirin or another NSAID or a steroid medication. Sedatives and tranquilizers can help control jerky movements.

Vasculitis

Vasculitis is the inflammation of a blood vessel. There are many types of vasculitis, and most are quite rare. Two of the more common types are described here.

Giant cell arteritis

If you develop new headaches, your temples are tender or painful and you're over 50 years old, you may have giant cell arteritis (ahr-tuh-RY-tis). This is an inflammation in the lining of your arteries, the blood vessels that carry oxygen-rich blood from your heart to the rest of your body. Giant cell arteritis (GCA) may also be associated with symptoms of arthritis — pain and stiffness in your neck, arms or hips.

Although GCA can affect the arteries in your neck, upper body and arms, it occurs most often in the arteries in your head and especially in your temples (temporal arteries). For this reason, the disorder is also known as temporal arteritis or cranial arteritis.

Older adults are at greatest risk of giant cell arteritis. About 200 of every 100,000 people over age 50 develop the disorder, making it the most common vasculitis in this group. On average, it occurs at age 70. Women are more likely than men to get this disease. People who have another inflammatory disease called polymyalgia rheumatica are also at greater risk of getting giant cell arteritis. The two disorders are closely linked — about half of people with GCA also have polymyalgia rheumatica. (For more information about polymyalgia rheumatica, see page 73.)

As with other autoimmune disorders, the inflammation of blood vessels in GCA stems from an abnormal immune system response. Exactly what causes this isn't known, but researchers believe that both genetic factors and aging play a role, along with some triggering factor.

Signs and symptoms. GCA frequently causes headaches, weight loss, fevers and fatigue. About two-thirds of people with GCA have a new, severe headache. Other signs and symptoms include:

- Sudden, painless partial or complete loss of vision in one or both eyes. Transient loss of vision or double vision may precede permanent vision loss.
- A tender, thickened artery in your temple.
- Scalp tenderness.
- Jaw pain when you chew (claudication).
- Throat or tongue pain.
- New pain and stiffness in your shoulders, neck, arms or hips, which is usually worse in the morning and improves with activity.

Left untreated, narrowed or blocked arteries can lead to permanent blindness, a stroke or an aneurysm.

Diagnosis. To diagnose GCA, your doctor may order blood tests, including an erythrocyte sedimentation rate and C-reactive protein test. These test results are usually highly elevated. An X-ray test of your large arteries (arteriogram) may be needed in some cases if signs and symptoms suggest that arteries in the arms and neck are affected. To confirm the diagnosis, a small sample (biopsy) may be taken of the temporal artery to be examined under the microscope. If you have GCA, the artery usually shows signs of inflammation, and large cells, called giant cells, which give the disease its name.

Treatment. Treatment of GCA consists of high doses (40 to 60 milligrams) of a corticosteroid drug such as prednisone. (These medications are discussed on page 94.) Because GCA can cause vision loss, immediate treatment is necessary. Your doctor may start this medication even before confirming the diagnosis by way of a biopsy. You may need to continue taking steroid medications for two years or longer. After the first month, the dosage may gradually be lowered until you reach the lowest dose needed to control inflammation.

In addition to corticosteroids, you may take a low dose (80 to 100 milligrams) of aspirin each day to reduce the risk of complications.

Polymyalgia rheumatica

Polymyalgia rheumatica (pol-ee-my-AL-juh roo-MA-ti-kah) (PMR) is an inflammatory disorder that affects the same group of people as giant cell arteritis (see page 71) does. But polymyalgia rheumatica is more common than giant cell arteritis.

The term *polymyalgia rheumatica* comes from the Greek words that mean "pain in many muscles." It causes widespread muscle aching and joint stiffness, especially in your neck, shoulders, thighs and hips. Inflammation may develop elsewhere in your body as well.

PMR is about as common as rheumatoid arthritis, affecting about 1 percent of older people. The disease is rarely seen in people under age 50. Women are more likely than men to develop PMR, and people of northern European and Scandinavian descent are at higher risk.

Just what triggers PMR isn't known, but aging and genetic and environmental factors probably all play a role.

Signs and symptoms. PMR is characterized by pain and stiffness in the muscles of your shoulders, neck, upper arms, lower back, thighs and hips. Stiffness is usually worse in the morning or after sitting or lying down for long periods. A slight fever, fatigue and unexplained weight loss may also occur.

Symptoms may come on abruptly or gradually. People with the condition may go to bed feeling fine, only to awaken in pain the next morning. Others may develop a worsening of aching, stiffness and fatigue over weeks or longer.

People with PMR may also have giant cell arteritis either before or after having PMR. The two disorders can also occur at the same time.

Diagnosis. If your symptoms suggest the possibility of polymyalgia rheumatica, your doctor may order blood tests. The sed rate is usually elevated in people with PMR. The rheumatoid factor test can help rule out a diagnosis of rheumatoid arthritis, since rheumatoid factor isn't usually present in people with PMR.

Treatment. NSAIDs such as aspirin and ibuprofen can be effective for mild symptoms. The usual treatment, however, is a low, daily dose of a corticosteroid drug, which generally provides immediate and complete relief from symptoms. PMR usually goes away after a year or two.

Polyarteritis nodosa

Polyarteritis nodosa (pol-e-ahr-tuh-RI-tis no-DOH-suh), or PAN, is a type of vasculitis, or inflammation of the blood vessel system — your veins, arteries and capillaries. Although less common than giant cell arteritis (discussed on page 71), polyarteritis nodosa is a serious and sometimes fatal disorder that involves inflammation of many arteries, especially small and medium-sized ones.

PAN can affect many sites in the body. The skin, intestines, kidneys, nerves and heart are at greatest risk. The inflammation of PAN may cause blockage of the arteries, reducing the supply of blood to affected areas.

Polyarteritis nodosa can affect people of any age, including children, but middle-aged men are most likely to develop it. The causes of PAN are unknown, though some cases are caused by the hepatitis B virus.

Signs and symptoms. Symptoms of PAN include fever, muscle pain or weakness, weight loss, fatigue and joint aches and pains. You may have tingling, numbness or pain in your hands, arms, feet and legs. Skin problems, such as rashes or sores, are common. Many people with PAN have high blood pressure. If the intestines are involved, you may have abdominal pain and bloody diarrhea.

Diagnosis. If your symptoms suggest that you may have PAN, your doctor will do a biopsy of a sample of tissue affected by the arteritis, such as your skin, muscle or a nerve. The biopsy can show changes in small or medium-sized arteries that occur in the disease. Your doctor may also order an X-ray test (angiogram) of abdominal or other blood vessels. Blood tests may also be useful. The sedimentation rate is usually elevated in PAN.

Treatment. Left untreated, polyarteritis nodosa is often fatal. With early diagnosis and proper treatment, however, the disease can be controlled. Many people with PAN lead normal lives.

Treatment includes high doses of a corticosteroid drug such as prednisone in combination with an immunosuppressant medication such as cyclophosphamide, which slows down immune system activity. You'll find more information about corticosteroids and immunosuppressants in Chapter 5, which covers medications for arthritis.

Moving forward

Even though inflammatory arthritic and connective tissue disorders are chronic diseases, you may be able to avoid their most severe consequences and lead an active, productive life. Both professional care and self-care are essential.

By following a carefully planned, individualized treatment program outlined by your doctor and other health care professionals, many people find that they can reduce the impact of these diseases. Diet, exercise and knowing when to stop and rest are all elements in this approach to successfully managing your condition.

Part 2

Treating arthritis

Chapter 5

Medications for arthritis

Just as there's a spectrum of symptoms among people with various forms of arthritis, a broad range of medications is available to help control pain and slow or prevent joint damage. You and your doctor have many options.

Medications can help relieve your pain, make movement easier and prevent further damage from inflammation. Some medications are sold without a prescription and are common enough to be sold in convenience stores. Others are powerful prescription-only drugs. Some are used to treat several forms of arthritis, while others are used for a particular type.

Medications can help you feel better and allow you to lead a more active life. Like all drugs, though, arthritis medications can cause side effects, ranging from dry mouth to an upset stomach to an increased risk of infection, heart attack or stroke. The benefits of these drugs must be weighed against potentially dangerous side effects. Only you and your doctor can determine how the known risks of a particular drug stack up against the benefits for you.

For most people with arthritis, medications play an important role in a treatment plan that also includes nondrug therapies and lifestyle modifications. In the past, rheumatoid arthritis and other forms of the disease were considered disabling and difficult to manage. New medications and combinations of treatments have made arthritis a treatable disease and have greatly improved quality of life and outlook for many people.

Different drugs, different uses

Your doctor may recommend one or more over-the-counter (OTC) or prescription medications, depending on your type of arthritis, how much pain you have and other factors.

If you have osteoarthritis, you may benefit from medications, particularly for pain relief. For mild to moderate pain, acetaminophen (Tylenol, others) is often effective. For moderate to severe pain, and if you have signs of inflammation, you might take nonsteroidal anti-inflammatory drugs (NSAIDs), such as aspirin, naproxen or ibuprofen. Other types of pain relievers, including topical creams, gels, ointments and sprays, may also help. Some people with osteoarthritis benefit from injections of corticosteroid drugs or hyaluronic acid (similar to natural joint fluid) directly into affected joints.

If you have rheumatoid arthritis, suppressing inflammation is especially important because of the damage it can cause. Controlling inflammation also helps reduce pain. Medications are also used to help control the underlying immune system abnormalities in rheumatoid arthritis and slow or stop damage to joints. Joint damage can happen early-on in rheumatoid arthritis, so many doctors begin aggressive treatment quickly, often using a combination of drugs.

There are six primary groups of medications that doctors recommend for arthritis. Some drugs have properties that allow them to fit into more than one category. These groups are:

- Analgesics
- Nonsteroidal anti-inflammatory drugs
- Corticosteroids, also called glucocorticoids or steroids
- Disease-modifying antirheumatic drugs (DMARDs)
- Immunosuppressant drugs
- Biologic agents

Other drugs may also be used to treat various forms of arthritis. For example, antidepressants in low doses can be helpful in treating pain.

Analgesic vs. anti-inflammatory
Although some drugs, such as aspirin and other NSAIDs, have both anti-inflammatory and analgesic effects, these two functions are different.

Analgesics relieve pain. Non-narcotic analgesics, such as acetaminophen and aspirin, are used for mild pain. Narcotic analgesics are available by prescription only and are generally reserved for the relief of severe pain that disrupts your quality of life. Many are potentially addictive.

Anti-inflammatory drugs (NSAIDs and corticosteroids) reduce the inflammation that can cause permanent damage to joints. Inflammation results in increased blood flow, which produces swelling, redness, pain and heat.

Pain reducers (analgesics)

When arthritis causes pain, you naturally want relief as quickly as possible. Analgesics, or painkillers, can provide that relief, but some come with serious side effects, including the potential for dependency. Your body may eventually develop a tolerance for painkillers, so the longer you take them, the less effective they are. In addition, by masking your pain, these drugs may fool you into thinking that you can be more active than you should be, leading to additional damage or injury.

The two most familiar nonaddictive analgesics are aspirin and acetaminophen. Aspirin has both analgesic and anti-inflammatory effects and may cause stomach irritation in some people. Acetaminophen (Tylenol, others) is an OTC pain reducer that isn't an NSAID. It's less likely than aspirin or other NSAIDs to irritate your stomach, but it has a limited effect on inflammation. Acetaminophen is appropriate for people whose arthritis causes pain but little inflammation — as is often the case in osteoarthritis — and for those who are unable to take NSAIDs.

Many people with arthritis find that acetaminophen can ease their discomfort as effectively as an NSAID can. In particular, if you have mild pain from osteoarthritis, rheumatologists recommend acetaminophen as the first choice for pain relief. It's inexpensive and usually doesn't cause side effects.

If needed, you can use an NSAID with acetaminophen for a short time. But don't take more than the recommended dose of acetaminophen, because it can lead to liver problems, especially if you consume three or more alcoholic drinks daily.

Although acetaminophen has generally been considered safe, some research suggests that taking daily doses of 500 milligrams (mg) or more may increase the risk of high blood pressure. In a study that examined the medical records of more than 5,000 women for up to eight years, those who took 500 mg or more of aceta-minophen a day were about twice as likely to develop high blood pressure as were women who didn't use the drug. These findings were the same whether the women used the medication for headache, arthritis, or other aches and pains. Researchers aren't sure why acetaminophen may raise blood pressure, but it's thought to influence blood vessel control.

An analgesic that is neither an NSAID nor a narcotic is tramadol (Ultram). For many people, this medication is effective for pain relief. It can be used alone or along with acetaminophen or an NSAID. Studies show that taking tramadol can allow you to take a lower dose of an NSAID and achieve the same level of pain control. If you don't want to or are unable to take an NSAID, tramadol can provide similar relief.

Side effects of tramadol may include nausea, loss of appetite, constipation, diarrhea, dizziness, drowsiness and increased sweat-ing. The drug can be habit-forming in people who have addictive tendencies.

For severe pain that isn't relieved by other medications, doctors sometimes prescribe narcotic analgesics. The strongest of these are derived from opium or are made synthetically to have opium-like characteristics. Some of these products also contain acetaminophen. Narcotics work by blocking pain signals that travel to the brain.

Because narcotics may cause dependency, they're prescribed mainly for short-term and intense pain. Some doctors use these drugs to treat chronic arthritis pain, being careful to monitor for possible dependency.

Narcotic painkillers include the following:

- Acetaminophen with codeine (Tylenol No. 2, 3, 4, Tylenol with Codeine Elixir)
- Codeine
- Hydrocodone with acetaminophen (Hydrocet, Lorcet, Lortab, Norco, Vicodin)
- Hydrocodone with ibuprofen (Vicoprofen)
- Meperidine (Demerol, Meperidine Hydrochloride)
- Morphine sulfate (Avinza, MSIR, MS Contin, Oramorph SR)
- Oxycodone (OxyContin, Roxicodone, OxyFAST, OxyIR, others)
- Oxycodone with acetaminophen (Endocet, Percocet, Roxicet, Tylox)
- Oxycodone with aspirin (Endodan, Percodan)
- Propoxyphene (Darvon, Darvon-N)
- Propoxyphene with acetaminophen (Darvocet-N)

NSAIDs

A main goal in treating rheumatoid arthritis, osteoarthritis and several other arthritic disorders is to stop inflammation. Inflammation can cause permanent damage to the affected areas, as well as pain and discomfort.

Two main categories of anti-inflammatory medications are used by people with arthritis. One contains cortisone, or cortisone-related substances, such as prednisone or methylprednisolone. These substances — known as corticosteroids, glucocorticoids or steroids — are synthetic forms of cortisol, a natural hormone in your body. Corticosteroids can control inflammation effectively. But if you take them for a long time, they may cause serious side effects.

The other category of anti-inflammatory drugs has no steroids. These medications go by the name nonsteroidal anti-inflammatory drugs, or NSAIDs. They range from the most widely used drug in the world — aspirin — to over-the-counter products such as ibuprofen to more potent NSAIDs available only with a prescription. Whatever type of arthritis you have, you're likely to have taken an NSAID at some point.

There are several classes of NSAIDS. Those used to treat arthritis may be divided into three groups:

- Salicylates, including aspirin
- Traditional NSAIDs, such as ibuprofen (Advil, Motrin, others) and naproxen (Naprelan)
- COX-2 inhibitors — celecoxib (Celebrex)

Long-term use of NSAIDs has been called into question in recent years because of concerns about serious side effects — in particular, potentially life-threatening stomach and intestinal bleeding and a possible increased risk of heart attack, stroke and other cardiovascular problems. If you're using NSAIDs to manage your arthritis, talk to your doctor about the risks and benefits of these drugs for your particular situation. (See "Drug worries — Weighing the risks and benefits," page 92.) Don't stop any drug regime without talking to your doctor first.

How NSAIDs work

NSAIDs work in two ways. They relieve pain and fever, and they reduce swelling and inflammation. Certain NSAIDs, such as aspirin, buffered aspirin and ibuprofen, are used for relief of everyday pain. If you have osteoarthritis, you may take NSAIDs in small doses to reduce pain. These painkillers also help relieve other common aches and pains, such as headaches and menstrual cramps.

If you have rheumatoid arthritis, NSAIDs are valuable because of their ability to reduce the joint pain, stiffness and swelling caused by inflammation. Despite minor differences between types of NSAIDs, they all work against inflammation in a similar way. NSAIDs inhibit an enzyme called cyclooxygenase (COX). This enzyme promotes the production of prostaglandins, hormone-like chemicals in the blood and tissues that help send pain messages to the brain and are key to the process of inflammation.

In general, larger doses of NSAIDs are needed to reduce inflammation than are needed for pain relief. If you have osteoarthritis, you can usually take a smaller dose of an NSAID, because inflammation isn't usually severe and the pain comes and goes. But if you have rheumatoid arthritis, you'll probably need to take larger doses of an NSAID to achieve an anti-inflammatory effect.

Choosing an NSAID

Many different NSAIDs, both over-the-counter and prescription medications, are used to treat arthritis. Traditional NSAIDs make up the largest group of drugs in this class, with about 20 prescription medications. Of those, three are available in nonprescription strengths and sold over the counter (see page 86).

Because every person with arthritis is different, the best choice of NSAID varies from individual to individual. What works for you may not work for your best friend, and vice versa. That's why you and your doctor will choose an NSAID on the basis of several criteria:

• Your age and state of health
• The type and severity of your arthritis
• The frequency of medication needed
• How you respond to a medication
• How your other medications may interact with the NSAID
• The cost of medications
• Your risk of adverse side effects

Often your doctor will start you with a less expensive, OTC NSAID such as ibuprofen or naproxen. If the first drug you try doesn't provide adequate relief, you can switch to another class of NSAID.

Because of the risk of side effects, your doctor will prescribe the lowest effective dose of an NSAID for the shortest time possible, or only as needed.

Over-the-counter NSAIDs

Aspirin and its variants come in a range of dosages and in several forms — tablet, coated tablet, capsule, chewable tablet, effervescent tablet, gum and suppository. Buffered and coated types reduce potential stomach irritation and acidity. Some common OTC brand-name aspirins include Bayer and Bufferin. Many generic forms are also available.

A relatively small dose of aspirin (two 325-milligram tablets every four hours) usually suffices for everyday pain relief. That's how someone with osteoarthritis might use it.

Although aspirin can relieve pain from rheumatoid arthritis, it generally must be taken in frequent high doses — nine to 15 ordinary aspirin tablets in a day. This often causes serious side effects such as gastrointestinal bleeding and kidney problems. For this reason, many doctors advise people with rheumatoid arthritis to use other types of NSAIDs instead.

Three traditional NSAIDs are available in nonprescription strengths:

- Ibuprofen (Advil, Motrin IB, others)
- Ketoprofen (Orudis KT)
- Naproxen sodium (Aleve)

In 2005, the Food and Drug Administration (FDA) asked manufacturers of over-the-counter NSAIDs (not including aspirin and related drugs) to provide information to consumers about a possible increased risk of cardiovascular problems and serious gastrointestinal bleeding, as well as potential skin reactions. (See "NSAID side effects" on page 88.)

Prescription NSAIDs

Many NSAIDs, including some that contain aspirin, are available only with a prescription. In general, prescription NSAIDs come in higher doses than do OTC drugs.

With some prescription NSAIDs, you take just one or two doses a day. Beyond their convenience, these products can help ensure that you take your medication properly. Sometimes, it's hard to remember to take all your medications if you use more than one.

One-a-day NSAIDs include:

- Diclofenac sodium (Voltaren XR)
- Etodolac (Lodine XL)
- Ketoprofen (Oruvail)
- Meloxicam (Mobic)
- Nabumetone (Relafen)
- Naproxen (Naprelan)
- Oxaprozin (Daypro)
- Piroxicam (Feldene)

Other prescription NSAIDs are prescribed in dosages of more than one a day. Here are some examples:

- Diclofenac with misoprostol (Arthrotec) — one tablet two to four times a day

---

Generic vs. brand name

Many drugs used for treating arthritis are available as both brand-name and generic medications. What's the difference?

A drug that's discovered or developed in a laboratory begins with a generic name selected by experts and governmental agencies. Then the company that developed it typically gives it a brand name and sells it exclusively for a fixed period, usually 20 years. When those patent rights expire, any other drug company can manufacture and sell the drug under its generic name or another brand name. In any case, the Food and Drug Administration still must approve it.

Generic versions are available for almost half of all drugs on the market. For consumers, that's good news because generics often cost considerably less than their brand-name counterparts. Generic drugs have the same active ingredients, strength and dosage form as the brand-name versions. They also carry the same risks and benefits.

You, your doctor and pharmacist can determine whether you should use a brand-name medication or a generic version, based on your medical needs and ability to afford the medication.

- Fenoprofen calcium — one or two capsules three to four times a day
- Flurbiprofen (Ansaid) — one tablet two to four times a day
- Indomethacin (Indocin, Indocin SR) — one capsule two to four times a day
- Ketoprofen (Orudis) — one capsule three to four times a day
- Naproxen (Naprosyn) — one tablet twice a day
- Sulindac (Clinoril) — one tablet twice a day
- Tolmetin sodium (Tolectin, Tolectin DS) — one tablet three times a day

Nonacetylated salicylates are related to aspirin, but they tend to be gentler on the stomach and kidneys. They have only a minimal effect on the promotion of bleeding — a common side effect of NSAIDs. Prescription nonacetylated salicylates include choline and magnesium trisalicylates and salsalate (Mono-Gesic).

NSAID side effects

Most people who use NSAIDs for arthritis don't have problems, or they have minor side effects that resolve themselves. Side effects that may occur when you start using NSAIDs include:

- Mild headache
- Lightheadedness
- Drowsiness
- Dizziness

Reduce your risk of stomach problems from NSAIDs

NSAIDs can make your life easier by helping control the pain and inflammation of arthritis. Unfortunately, they can also give you an upset stomach or even an ulcer.

Gastrointestinal bleeding is a potentially serious side effect of NSAIDs. In addition to suppressing the prostaglandins that are associated with inflammation and pain, NSAIDs decrease production of a prostaglandin that protects your stomach lining. This allows gastric acid to erode the lining and cause bleeding and ulcers. A type of bacteria called *Helicobacter pylori* causes almost two-thirds of all ulcers. Most other ulcers are caused by NSAIDs.

Because stomach ulcers or bleeding can occur with no warning, it's important to get regular checkups. If you're taking NSAIDs regularly, your blood counts and liver enzymes should be checked periodically. Your doctor may also suggest that you take a medication to decrease some of the gastrointestinal side effects.

Histamine blockers, such as famotidine (Pepcid), cimetidine (Tagamet) and ranitidine (Zantac), and proton pump inhibitors such as omeprazole (Prilosec) and lansoprazole (Prevacid), reduce the amount of acid produced by your stomach. A drug called misoprostol (Cytotec) replaces the prostaglandin that protects the stomach. Proton pump inhibitors and misoprostol can decrease the risk of getting an ulcer. Some drugs are combinations of misoprostol and an NSAID.

The enzyme suppressed by NSAIDs, cyclooxygenase, has two forms, COX-1 and COX-2. Part of the role of COX-1 is to protect your stomach lining. Suppressing COX-1 can result in stomach

These effects are apt to go away within a week or two. If they don't, tell your doctor. Ringing or noise in your ears (tinnitus) may occur if you're using aspirin or a related medication.

If you're using large doses of NSAIDs or take these drugs over a long period of time, you should be aware of the potential for more-serious side effects. These may include:

- Stomach and intestinal irritation, such as cramps, pain or discomfort, diarrhea, heartburn, indigestion, nausea or vomiting

problems and bleeding. A different class of NSAIDs, called COX-2 inhibitors, suppresses mainly the COX-2 enzyme, which is associated with inflammation and pain (see page 91). COX-2 inhibitors effectively relieve pain with a reduced risk of ulcers.

The only COX-2 inhibitor currently available in the United States is celecoxib (Celebrex). Other drugs in the class were withdrawn from the market after being linked to an increased risk of serious cardiovascular events, such as heart attack and stroke.

If you do take traditional NSAIDs, you can take some steps to minimize the risk of stomach problems:

- Take NSAIDs with food and water or milk.
- Avoid alcohol, since this increases the risk of gastric bleeding.
- Take the lowest possible dose you can to reduce symptoms.
- Take your medication later in the day if possible. If you take an NSAID once a day, doing so in the afternoon or evening may be easier on your stomach.
- Don't take more NSAIDs than prescribed or more often than prescribed.
- Don't take the drugs with other prescription or OTC NSAIDs.
- Talk to your doctor about any other medications you take that may interact with NSAIDs to increase your risk of stomach problems.

Acetaminophen (Tylenol, others) may be used instead of NSAIDs to reduce pain and fever without causing gastrointestinal side effects. Unlike the NSAIDs, however, it doesn't reduce inflammation.

Aspirin and NSAIDs

Many people take a low-dose daily aspirin to help prevent heart attack and stroke. Aspirin helps maintain blood flow to the heart by reducing the risk of blockages in the arteries. But for reasons that aren't clear, NSAIDs such as ibuprofen may counteract the benefit of daily aspirin therapy.

That doesn't mean you should stop taking aspirin. Studies indicate that it's still effective if taken two hours before a single daily dose of ibuprofen. But taking multiple doses of ibuprofen daily or taking ibuprofen before aspirin can impair the protective effect of aspirin. A recent study showed that occasional use of ibuprofen — less than 60 days a year — doesn't seem to impair aspirin's ability to reduce the risk of heart attack.

If you need only a single dose of ibuprofen, take it two hours after the aspirin. If you need to take ibuprofen or another traditional NSAID more often, talk to your doctor about medication alternatives.

- Gastrointestinal bleeding, including ulcers
- Increased sensitivity to sunlight
- Decreased kidney function
- Fluid retention
- Serious skin reactions
- High blood pressure
- Heart failure

NSAIDs have anti-clotting effects, so you may notice that you bleed or bruise more easily. Large doses of NSAIDs can also lead to kidney problems and fluid retention, which can worsen congestive heart failure. Mouth sores and skin rashes can occur while taking NSAIDs. If you have questions about symptoms that develop while taking an NSAID, talk with your doctor.

In addition to the known side effects, some research suggests that use of traditional NSAIDs may increase your risk of heart attack, stroke and other cardiovascular (CV) events. For example, a study of the NSAID naproxen for prevention of Alzheimer's disease raised concerns that it may be associated with an increased risk of heart attack. If there is an increased risk, it's likely small. It has not emerged as a concern in the roughly 30 years that the drug has been available.

Because of the possibility that other NSAIDs, such as ibuprofen, pose this same risk, in 2005 the FDA called for label changes on all over-the-counter and prescription NSAIDs. Manufacturers must include warnings about potential CV risks and rare but serious skin reactions from using these drugs. These label changes don't apply to aspirin because it has clearly been shown to reduce the risk of heart attack and stroke in certain people.

More studies are needed to determine whether the potential increased cardiovascular risk applies to everyone who uses NSAIDs or just to people who also have other risk factors for cardiovascular disease. In addition, researchers don't know exactly what level of NSAID use increases this risk. The results of preliminary studies conflict with data from earlier research on the same drugs. Most people who are doing well with these drugs can continue to take them.

The risks of adverse side effects are higher in older adults, especially women, and in people with other medical conditions. If you've had stomach ulcers, gastrointestinal bleeding or kidney failure, or if you're taking a blood thinner (anticoagulant) or a platelet aggregation inhibitor such as clopidogrel (Plavix), your doctor probably won't recommend traditional NSAIDs. People who have just had coronary bypass surgery or recently had a stroke or transient ischemic attacks (TIAs) also should avoid these drugs.

Side effects of NSAIDs tend to be worse if you're taking more than one NSAID or if you also take oral corticosteroids. Drug interactions can occur if you take NSAIDs and also take an oral diabetes medication, beta blocker or diuretic. Tell your doctor about all other medications you use, including herbal preparations.

COX-2 inhibitors

This class of medications is similar to NSAIDs, but the drugs work in a different manner. COX-2 inhibitors were developed with the

---

Drug worries — Weighing the risks and benefits

First rofecoxib (Vioxx) was pulled from the market in 2004 with no advance notice after a large cancer-prevention study found a statistically increased risk of heart attack and stroke in study participants treated with Vioxx, as compared with a placebo. A few months later, valdecoxib (Bextra) was withdrawn because of unanswered questions about its cardiovascular safety.

Warnings also emerged about potential cardiovascular risks of celecoxib (Celebrex), naproxen (Aleve) and other nonsteroidal anti-inflammatory drugs. This unsettling news left many people with arthritis wondering where to turn. What if you rely on these drugs to relieve joint pain and stiffness, but fear heart problems if you continue to take them?

First, take a step back and realize that you have several options for pain control. Traditional NSAIDs or the available COX-2 inhibitor may continue to play a role in managing arthritis pain for many people. But a variety of other drug and non-drug therapies can also help.

When taking any medication, it's important to evaluate the benefits and risks. All drugs — including "natural" and herbal remedies and supplements — can have side effects, and most if not all drugs pose some risk. Doctors prescribe drugs when they

---

aim of reducing some of the well-recognized side effects of traditional NSAIDs. But COX-2 inhibitors appear to be associated with an increased risk of cardiovascular problems.

Like traditional NSAIDs, COX-2 inhibitors block the production of cyclooxygenase, an enzyme that produces prostaglandins — the hormone-like substances that trigger inflammation and pain. But unlike NSAIDs, COX-2 inhibitors mainly affect only one of the two forms of COX, instead of both.

The two forms of COX have separate functions:

- **COX-1.** This form produces prostaglandins that help maintain kidney blood flow, protect your stomach against harmful acid that can erode its lining, and allow blood platelets to function normally in clotting blood.

believe the benefits outweigh the risks. Often this means accepting some risk. Penicillin, for example, carries a risk of allergic
reaction. For most people, the risk is small but real — and, in the
face of a raging infection, is clearly outweighed by the benefits.
For people with a history of a significant penicillin allergy, the
risk may be high enough to warrant using a different therapy.

To make that judgment, doctors need to know about the relative risks of different forms of therapy, the groups of people
who may be at highest risk and the potential alternatives. The
goal is to find the option that provides the lowest risk and
greatest benefit.

So it is with anti-inflammatory drugs. Their benefits are
important for many people. At this point, the risks are not clearly defined. Different studies, none of them designed to look
specifically at cardiovascular risk, have produced conflicting
data. Without evidence from clinical trials designed to show
how Celebrex or Aleve might affect cardiovascular risk in the
general population, doctors have to use their best clinical judgment, recognizing that there is no one-size-fits-all solution.
Together you and your doctor can make an informed decision
about how best to treat your arthritis.

- **COX-2.** This form of the enzyme contributes to the
  development of prostaglandins associated with pain and
  inflammation.

When researchers realized that traditional NSAIDs blocked both
versions of the COX enzyme, the quest was on for a more selective
pain reliever — one that would block pain, yet not harm your gastrointestinal lining. This research led to the development of COX-2
inhibitors. The first COX-2 inhibitor was approved by the FDA
in 1999.

In clinical studies, COX-2 inhibitors were shown to relieve joint
pain just as well as traditional NSAIDs, but they caused fewer
ulcers and less gastrointestinal bleeding. However, data from later
clinical trials showed that COX-2 inhibitors may increase the risk of

serious cardiovascular problems, such as heart attack or stroke, especially when used in high doses or for long periods in people with existing CV disease.

As a result, two popular COX-2 inhibitors, rofecoxib (Vioxx) and valdecoxib (Bextra), were withdrawn from the market. The only COX-2 inhibitor currently available is the prescription drug celecoxib (Celebrex). Because of concerns that Celebrex, like Vioxx and Bextra, may pose an increased risk of heart attack and stroke, the FDA asked the drug manufacturer to revise its product label to include a warning of the medication's cardiovascular and gastrointestinal risks.

Side effects of COX-2 inhibitors are generally mild. They may include symptoms of respiratory infection, headache, dizziness, diarrhea, nausea, heartburn and stomach pain. These drugs can also cause kidney problems, high blood pressure and fluid retention. Although the risk of stomach bleeding is generally lower if you take Celebrex than if you take a traditional NSAID, it's important to realize that stomach bleeding can still occur. Older adults may be at higher risk of all of these side effects.

If you've experienced gastrointestinal problems from traditional NSAIDs — or are at high risk of such problems — Celebrex may be a safe and appropriate treatment for you. Celebrex also might be a good choice if you take drugs that contain the corticosteroid prednisone. Corticosteroids, like NSAIDs, can cause stomach bleeding. To take traditional NSAIDs on top of those drugs would further increase your risk of bleeding.

If you do take Celebrex, talk with your doctor about the lowest effective dose for the shortest duration possible.

Corticosteroids

Corticosteroids, also called steroids or glucocorticoids, are the second of the two major types of drugs used to fight inflammation in people with arthritis. Corticosteroids work by blocking your body's ability to make substances that can cause inflammation, such as prostaglandins.

Corticosteroids also serve another function for people with rheumatoid arthritis. In rheumatoid arthritis and other autoimmune diseases, your immune system mistakenly attacks healthy tissue instead of attacking invaders such as bacteria and viruses. Corticosteroids reduce autoimmune activity, lowering its potential to do harm. For example, the drugs cause white blood cells to work less effectively. Unfortunately, this means that the immune system's ability to fend off infection is also reduced to varying degrees in different people.

Corticosteroids are synthetic (artificial) versions of a hormone called cortisol. Cortisol is produced by your adrenal glands. It has many vital functions in your body. It helps regulate the balance of water and salt and your body's use (metabolism) of protein, fat and carbohydrates. During times of stress — such as an illness or a period of emotional upset — your adrenal glands excrete extra cortisol to help your body deal with the stress.

Although the names resemble each other, corticosteroids aren't the same as the anabolic steroids used by athletes to enhance their performance in competition. Anabolic steroids have no value in treating arthritis. In fact, the general term *steroid* refers to several related chemical substances, including many hormones, bile acids, natural drugs such as digitalis compounds, and the beginning forms (precursors) of some vitamins.

Corticosteroids became widely known more than a half-century ago, when scientists led by physicians and investigators at Mayo Clinic discovered them and began using them to treat arthritis, with remarkably positive results. At the time, it was thought that a cure was at hand for arthritis. But in succeeding years it became clear that because of their toxicity, corticosteroids couldn't be used in high doses for long periods. The side effects were sometimes worse than the symptoms of arthritis.

When corticosteroids are needed

If you have rheumatoid arthritis, your doctor may first turn to NSAIDs to control inflammation and provide you with some relief. But the NSAIDs you try might not be potent enough to reduce the inflammation, or they may cause undesirable side effects.

Medication half-life

The amount of time needed to eliminate a drug from the body depends on a number of factors, such as the drug's rate of clearance from circulation by the kidneys or liver, and which tissues the drug penetrates or binds to. The term *half-life* refers to the amount of time required to eliminate or decrease the blood concentration of a drug by one-half. The half-life is a standard way to measure how long a drug stays in the body. The half-life of different drugs varies a great deal and can be used as a guide to determine how frequently a drug should be given. For example, a medication with a short half-life needs to be taken at more frequent intervals than a drug with a long half-life.

Some medications have very short half-lives. For two ibuprofen tablets, the half-life is about two hours. Plain aspirin has a half-life of about four hours. But some nonsteroidal anti-inflammatory drugs, such as piroxicam (Feldene), have a half-life of 50 hours or so. Gold (a disease-modifying antirheumatic drug) can have a half-life of up to three or four months when multiple doses are taken.

Corticosteroids fight inflammation effectively and quickly. They ease symptoms of stiffness, pain and fatigue, and they reduce swelling, helping protect your joints. If other tissues are involved, such as eyes and internal organs, inflammation is also reduced and they're protected from damage. In the short term, corticosteroids can make you feel dramatically better.

For many people, corticosteroids are needed only occasionally to relieve acute symptoms or during a flare. For others, a low dose of a corticosteroid may be needed for long periods of time. If you have severe arthritis that affects several joints, a corticosteroid, often prednisone, can be taken by mouth to treat widespread inflammation. In both osteoarthritis and rheumatoid arthritis, cortisone can be injected directly into the inflamed joint. (See "Joint injections" on page 98.)

Given the serious side effects, use of corticosteroids in treating arthritis depends very much on their effective and safe management. In other words, your doctor needs to devise a treatment plan that not only works but also keeps side effects to an absolute minimum.

Another steroid medication — adrenocorticotropic hormone (ACTH), the pituitary hormone that stimulates the adrenal glands to secrete cortisol — is no longer used in treating arthritis.

Short-term therapy

Some people with arthritis need quick relief of their symptoms. For instance, they may have a flare-up that's painful, incapacitating or potentially damaging. If this happens to you, your doctor may put you on a short course of corticosteroids (steroid taper), which commonly produces relief in a matter of a few days. It may also be used to tide you over — allowing you to feel better and reduce damage while you wait for other medications to become effective.

With a short course of corticosteroids, you begin with a moderate dose of the drug. Then, every few days after that, you take a smaller and smaller dose. This approach minimizes the possibility of side effects. To simplify matters, special packages are available that follow the doses of the steroid taper exactly. You need only take the doses indicated, day by day, throughout the specified period. This drug therapy may last a week or two.

Because of the significant amounts of corticosteroids used in steroid tapers, they shouldn't be used very often. Corticosteroid injections can also be used as a short-term approach to treating rheumatoid arthritis.

Long-term therapy

Using a corticosteroid, such as prednisone, over a long period at doses of more than 10 milligrams daily, almost always produces significant side effects. But people with severe, unremitting rheumatoid arthritis may take low-dose corticosteroids for months to years at a time to keep the disease under control. The possibility of side effects is reduced with low doses, but side effects do occur.

In people who've recently developed rheumatoid arthritis, a low-dose course of corticosteroids is often used in combination with a disease-modifying antirheumatic drug (DMARD). The

Joint injections

When other methods such as NSAIDs, lifestyle approaches, disease-modifying antirheumatic drugs or even low doses of oral corticosteroids fail to ease the pain caused by rheumatoid arthritis, injection of corticosteroids in one or more joints is another option. This can dramatically reduce inflammation in one or several areas of your body, such as a knee or an elbow.

Relief may last for months, allowing a break in the cycle of inflammation and injury. If injections work well for you, they may be used again in the future. If there's no significant relief — or if it lasts only briefly — then injections aren't for you.

Some people with osteoarthritis and accompanying inflammation also may be helped by corticosteroid injections. Corticosteroids in oral form aren't considered appropriate for osteoarthritis. Oral medications affect the entire body, while injections tend to work primarily at the injection site. Corticosteroid injections also may be helpful if you have psoriatic arthritis, gout, tendinitis or bursitis.

Joint injections are usually performed at your doctor's office. A numbing agent (local anesthetic) is used to make the shot less painful. The corticosteroid is then injected into the joint space. The numbing agent wears off in a few hours. It may take a few days before the corticosteroid starts to work. In the interim, the injection site might be a little sore and swollen. An ice pack can help relieve symptoms.

Although corticosteroid injections generally don't have serious side effects, doctors limit the number of injections you can have within a given time period. Numerous injections in the same area of your body may damage the tissues they come into contact with.

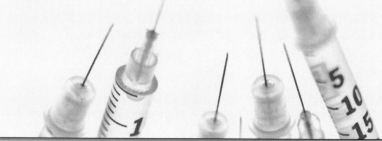

steroid provides relief until the DMARD begins to take effect, which could be a period of months. If the DMARD helps you, the dose of the corticosteroid can eventually be tapered and then use of the drug discontinued completely. Alternatively, your doctor may prescribe a low-dose corticosteroid and DMARD together for an indefinite period, especially if the DMARD doesn't work as hoped.

For long-term use, your doctor may prescribe a daily dose of about 5 to 10 mg of prednisone, or an equivalent dose of a similar drug. Another approach when you're receiving long-term therapy is to alternate the dose you take every few days. You may have a higher dose on day one and a lower dose on day two. The anti-inflammatory effect of the drug may not be as effective on the day the lower dose is taken. But if the effect does persist, your body gets the benefit of a low-dose day. Tapering from use of a low dose may take months or years.

Even at small doses, it's vital that you carefully follow your doctor's directions for taking corticosteroids. Any changes you make in the way that you take your medication can lead to potentially dangerous side effects. It's especially important to go off these medications gradually rather than all at once.

Corticosteroids by name

There are several different types of corticosteroids. Your doctor will select the type that's most appropriate for you. Some common corticosteroids are:
- Betamethasone (Celestone, Celestone Soluspan)
- Cortisone acetate
- Dexamethasone (Decadron)
- Hydrocortisone (Cortef)
- Methylprednisolone (Depo-Medrol, Medrol, Solu-Medrol)
- Prednisolone (Prelone)
- Prednisone (Sterapred)
- Triamcinolone (Aristocort, Kenalog)

Corticosteroids are available in both brand names and less costly generic versions. They come in several forms, including capsules and tablets, liquids for injection, as topical creams and in syrup for children.

Corticosteroid side effects

With small doses of corticosteroids — 7.5 milligrams (mg) or less of prednisone or the equivalent — the risk of side effects is reduced. Intermediate doses of 7.5 to 20 mg a day for a month are associated with a moderate risk. High doses of 20 to 60 mg involve a higher risk and should be taken only when absolutely required. Very high doses — 100 to 1,000 mg a day — are used very rarely and briefly.

Corticosteroids have many side effects — ranging from very common to rare. Some common side effects include:

- Weight gain from water retention
- Weight gain from increase in body fat, partly due to increased appetite
- Mood swings
- Nervousness
- Sleeplessness
- Easy bruising
- Slow healing of wounds
- Acne
- Development of a round face
- Blurred vision
- Weakness in arm or leg muscles
- Thinning hair or excessive hair growth
- Osteoporosis (thinning of bones)

Side effects that are most likely to happen only if you use moderate or high doses of corticosteroids include:

- Increased blood sugar level
- High blood pressure
- Stomach ulcers or irritation, usually when NSAIDs also are being taken
- Purple or red stretch marks on the skin
- Increased risk of infections

Some people are more susceptible to the risks of even small doses of corticosteroids. Older adults are more apt to have trouble than younger people are.

If you take high doses of corticosteroids, you may develop a dependency on the drug, because the high doses can cause your adrenal glands to stop making cortisol. If you've been taking corti-

Drug interactions

Many people use more than one medication, which may be pre-scribed to them by different physicians — specialists as well as a primary care doctor. They may also use OTC drugs. Unfortunately, the action of one drug can be altered by the action of another, either canceling out the desired effect or pro-ducing a dangerous reaction. Even OTC drugs can cause seri-ous interactions with prescription drugs.

When you take medications for arthritis, be sure to tell your doctor about every medication you use, including nonprescrip-tion medications, vitamins and minerals, and herbal supple-ments and alternative remedies. Bring all of your current med-ications whenever you visit any physician. That way, proper dosages can be figured for both prescription and nonprescrip-tion drugs. If needed, your doctor or clinic can create a medi-cine calendar for you. This way, you can take the drugs you need to take, but minimize the chance of potentially dangerous interactions.

costeroids for a long time, your body can't make enough cortisol. This can lead to an adrenal crisis — a potentially fatal develop-ment. Such a crisis may occur:

- During a heart attack
- During and immediately after a surgical procedure
- During an illness
- While you're unconscious and unable to communicate that you're taking corticosteroids

If you're using corticosteroids for a long period, wear a medical alert bracelet or necklace or other medical identification. If you're unable to communicate during an adrenal crisis, medical personnel will know they need to give you an extra dose of corticosteroids.

During periods of physical stress — when you're sick, are hav-ing surgery or have been injured — you may need to take higher doses of your steroid medication to avoid problems. If you're scheduled for surgery, talk to your doctor about your medication dosage.

Drug interactions are also possible with corticosteroids. That's why it's important to inform your doctor of any other medications that you may be using. (See "Drug interactions" on page 101.) For example, if you take insulin for diabetes and also take the corticosteroid prednisone, you may need to take a higher dose of insulin while you're taking prednisone. Taking the immunosuppressant drug cyclosporine while taking prednisone may increase the chance of convulsions.

Prednisone can also change the effects of other drugs you're taking, or have its effects changed. Some of those other drugs include:

- Amphotericin B
- Estrogen drugs
- Oral contraceptives
- Phenobarbital
- Strong diuretics, such as furosemide (Lasix)
- Blood thinners, such as warfarin (Coumadin)

Disease-modifying antirheumatic drugs (DMARDs)

Anti-inflammatory medications such as NSAIDs are valuable because they repress the inflammation that can damage your joints. But they do little to affect the basic disease process. To slow disease progression, doctors often turn to a class of medications called disease-modifying antirheumatic drugs, or DMARDs (DEE-mards). They're also sometimes called remittive or slow-acting drugs. They work by slowing down or suppressing your immune system.

DMARDs are most commonly used in the early stages of rheumatoid arthritis. Research shows that joint inflammation can cause irreversible damage early in the course of the disease — within two years of diagnosis. DMARDs may also be used for other inflammatory rheumatic diseases, including juvenile arthritis, ankylosing spondylitis, psoriatic arthritis and systemic lupus erythematosus.

Aggressive use of DMARDs as early as possible may help slow the disease and save your joints and other tissue from permanent damage. Early intervention with DMARDs can also improve longevity and quality of life.

DMARDs act slowly — they take several weeks or months to begin working. For this reason, doctors typically prescribe an NSAID or corticosteroid drug to ease your symptoms and control inflammation while the DMARD goes to work.

If your doctor prescribes DMARDs for you, you'll likely take more than one of these medications. Studies have shown that a combination of disease-modifying drugs provides more benefits than taking just one of these drugs — with no added side effects. Often three DMARDs are combined (known as "combination therapy" or "triple therapy").

There are several DMARDs that your doctor may consider:
• Hydroxychloroquine (Plaquenil)
• Gold (Myochrysine, Ridaura)
• Sulfasalazine (Azulfidine)
• Minocycline (Dynacin, Minocin)

Other forms of DMARDs include immunosuppressants, discussed on page 106, and biologic agents, which are covered on page 113.

Hydroxychloroquine

Among DMARDs, hydroxychloroquine (Plaquenil) has a reputation for having relatively few side effects. Originally a treatment for malaria, the medication has been on the market for many years. Hydroxychloroquine is thought to affect the way immune system cells work, taming the disease process. The medication is also used to treat systemic lupus erythematosus, psoriatic arthritis and other rheumatic diseases.

Hydroxychloroquine has to be taken daily in a dose of one or two tablets. You may be able to take a two-tablet dose at the same time. The medication can take up to three months to begin working and even longer to provide its full benefit. Its relative lack of side effects relieves you of the need for frequent blood tests and doctor's visits.

Although side effects are uncommon, they may include an upset stomach and rash. A rare effect is muscular weakness. A major side effect — which also occurs rarely — is damage to the eyes. Exposure to bright sunlight may increase the odds of this side effect occurring. If you take hydroxychloroquine, wear sunglasses and a broad-brimmed hat when you're outside on a sunny day. You'll also need to have your eyes checked by an ophthalmologist every six to 12 months.

Gold compounds

Gold-based drugs have been used to treat rheumatoid arthritis for decades. The form of gold used in medications is actually a gold salt and not the metal used in jewelry.

Gold has potent anti-inflammatory effects and slows joint damage, although exactly how it works isn't known. Half or more of people who take gold early in the development of their arthritis have good results. But gold compounds can cause dangerous side effects, and treatment with these drugs requires regular, close supervision from a physician. For this reason, gold-based medications aren't used as often as they once were.

At the start of a possible course of gold therapy, your doctor will begin by giving you a test dose of the drug. If you don't have a bad reaction, you'll usually start on weekly gold therapy. The dose is small at the outset, then gradually is increased to a full dose. Typically, you'll continue to get a full dose once a week for about five months. Your physician then makes adjustments according to your needs. The frequency may be reduced after several months.

Gold is administered two ways. You can take it as an injection in your buttock or as a capsule. You and your doctor will decide which is the best method for you.

Gold thiomalate (Myochrysine) is an injectable gold solution. Although an injection is likely to produce more positive results compared to gold in capsule form, that benefit is balanced by the inconvenience of visiting the doctor's office and the discomfort of the procedure. Your blood and urine also must be tested at the same time.

Auranofin (Ridaura) is oral gold, given in a daily dose of one or two capsules. In addition to avoiding the discomfort of a weekly injection, this form of gold also requires less frequent monitoring of blood and urine — perhaps just once a month. Auranofin produces fewer side effects but is generally not as effective as injectable gold.

Gold therapy is associated with three major side effects:
• Kidney damage
• Damage to bone marrow
• Rashes

Side effects can be serious. That's why you need to have your blood and urine tested regularly. Most side effects are mild and disappear when you stop taking the medication. Oral gold also may produce diarrhea. With injectable gold, joint pain may be worse for a few days, but it usually goes away after the first few injections.

Sulfasalazine

Sulfasalazine (Azulfidine) is similar to hydroxychloroquine in its effectiveness. Although originally developed as a treatment for rheumatoid arthritis, this medication is perhaps best known as an effective treatment of inflammatory bowel disease. Its ability to reduce inflammation seems to be due in part to an antibiotic effect on bacteria in the bowel. Sulfasalazine is also very effective in treating rheumatoid arthritis, and is widely used in treating both conditions.

If your doctor prescribes sulfasalazine, you'll probably begin with two 500-mg doses daily. If you don't experience troublesome side effects, your dose may be increased to 2 or 3 grams taken in two to four doses a day.

Sulfasalazine typically begins working more quickly than other DMARDs. Benefits may be noticeable after three to six weeks, although it may be longer.

Your doctor will order periodic blood tests to monitor the effect of the medication on your blood cells. Side effects are uncommon. Some people have stomach discomfort, which usually is eliminated by reducing the dose or by taking delayed-action (enteric-coated) tablets.

If you're allergic to sulfa or aspirin, don't take sulfasalazine. It's derived from sulfa and could cause an allergic reaction, such as a rash, asthma (wheezing), itching, fever or jaundice.

Minocycline

Minocycline (Dynacin, Minocin) is an antibiotic that can reduce swelling, tenderness and pain. Although it isn't approved by the

FDA for treatment of rheumatoid arthritis, minocycline is sometimes used "off label" for this purpose.

Minocycline has both an antibacterial action and works to inhibit the production of inflammatory cells that play a role in rheumatoid arthritis. Studies show a modest effect of the drug in preventing joint damage early in the disease. Like other DMARDs, minocycline takes weeks or even months to work.

Minocycline is often poorly tolerated. It may cause liver damage, as well as nausea, dizziness and a grayish skin discoloration. As with any antibiotic, this medication may lead to an overgrowth of germs that aren't affected by the drug. You might experience diarrhea, yeast infections or stomach distress.

Immunosuppressants

Because rheumatoid arthritis is thought to be an autoimmune disease, some medications are aimed at bringing the immune system under control. That's what immunosuppressant drugs do — they suppress or slow down the immune system. Some of these drugs are also cytotoxic, which means they attack and eliminate cells that are associated with rheumatoid arthritis. Immunosuppressants are usually considered a type of DMARD.

Several immunosuppressant drugs may be used by people with rheumatoid arthritis:

- Methotrexate (Rheumatrex, Trexall)
- Azathioprine (Imuran)
- Cyclosporine (Gengraf, Neoral)
- Cyclophosphamide (Cytoxan)
- Leflunomide (Arava)
- Mycophenolate (Cellcept)

Like most DMARDs, immunosuppressants can have major and potentially dangerous side effects. These medications can cause anemia and an increased risk of infection by reducing your body's ability to produce blood cells and suppressing the cells that are active in fighting infection. Some immunosuppressants seem to increase the likelihood of developing certain types of cancer after long-term use. Many can cause liver and kidney problems.

Side effects and allergies

The term *side effect* simply means a result of taking a medication (or receiving some other medical treatment) that occurs in addition to the primary and desired effect. Usually that means some unwanted, and possibly dangerous, effect. All drugs have some side effects.

Many medications used for arthritis treatment have a high potential for serious side effects. These drugs include corticosteroids, NSAIDs, DMARDs and immunosuppressants.

One possible side effect is a drug allergy. Not to be mistaken for an adverse drug reaction, drug allergies are a defective response by your immune system to a medication, just as you might have an allergic reaction to peanuts or plant pollen. Drug allergies show up in reactions that can be mild (a rash or hives), extremely serious (such as an anaphylactic reaction) or somewhere in between.

The discussion of side effects in this book is limited to some of the more important side effects and isn't intended to be complete. Your doctor can provide additional information on effects and side effects of the medications you're taking.

Women who want to become pregnant should avoid all immunosuppressants, especially methotrexate, cyclophosphamide, leflunomide and chlorambucil.

Methotrexate. Methotrexate (Rheumatrex, Trexall) is what's known as an antimetabolite drug. It does its job by blocking cells that generate some of the pain, inflammation and damage caused by rheumatoid arthritis. It also may slow the growth of synovial membrane cells lining the joint.

Methotrexate has been available for decades as a treatment for psoriasis and cancer. Since the 1980s, it's become the most popular DMARD for treating rheumatoid arthritis. The drug relieves symptoms and slows joint damage at all stages of the disease, and side effects are manageable. With its favorable risk-to-benefit profile and relatively low cost, methotrexate is the most commonly used DMARD in the United States.

Methotrexate is often combined with one or two other drugs, such as another DMARD. Using methotrexate as the cornerstone of combination therapy results in better control of rheumatoid arthritis than can be achieved with methotrexate alone, with no added side effects from combining medicines.

Methotrexate is taken by mouth, as tablets or liquid, and by injection. The liquid form is generally as effective as the tablet form and is cheaper. Methotrexate is typically taken in a single dose once a week.

It may not be appropriate for you to take methotrexate if:
- You're pregnant or plan to become pregnant
- You're breast-feeding
- You have medical problems such as kidney, liver or lung disease
- You're allergic to methotrexate
- You're taking any kind of prescription or OTC medications or supplements
- You're routinely exposed to people with colds and other infections
- You've been treated with X-rays or cancer drugs
- You use alcohol

Side effects vary from one person to another and may include:
- Nausea or stomach pain
- Diarrhea
- Fever, chills or general feeling of illness
- Headache
- Increased sun sensitivity
- Loss of appetite
- Hair loss
- Mouth ulcers or sores
- Rashes
- Lung inflammation
- Liver failure
- Anemia

Drugs such as methotrexate can also reduce the infection-fighting potency of your white blood cells, making you more vulnerable to infection. They can lower the number of platelets, so you bruise or bleed more easily, and cut down on your red blood cells, causing fatigue. If you notice these or any other side effects, contact your doctor.

If your doctor prescribes methotrexate, you'll need to have your blood tested regularly. This testing helps ensure that the drug doesn't produce any unwanted changes in your liver and bone marrow. Blood tests and visits with your doctor can help address any side effects in a timely manner. Many side effects can be managed by modifying the dose or manner of taking the drug or by taking folic acid along with the methotrexate.

Azathioprine. Azathioprine (Imuran) is used most commonly to protect kidney and heart transplants from being attacked and rejected by the body's immune system. Azathioprine holds white blood cells in check and can restrain the autoimmune effects that are part of rheumatoid arthritis. Of course, that also means that your body's ability to fight off infection is weakened.

Azathioprine isn't used often, but some doctors prescribe it for people who are taking a corticosteroid medication, so that the dose of the steroid can be reduced and eventually discontinued.

In addition to an increased vulnerability to infection, other side effects of azathioprine include:
- Gastrointestinal distress, such as heartburn, nausea and vomiting
- Bleeding and bruising more easily than normal
- Fatigue or weakness
- Loss of appetite
- Fevers and chills
- Increased risk of certain cancers

Your dosage is based on your body weight, and you take the medication with food. Your doctor will supervise your progress while you're taking azathioprine, including blood tests every few weeks.

It's particularly important to avoid taking azathioprine if you also take a gout drug called allopurinol (Zyloprim). The combination in your body adds to the toxic effect and, if used, requires special dosing and close supervision.

Cyclosporine. For the most part, cyclosporine (Gengraf, Neoral) has been used for people who have had organ transplants. It helps to prevent the immune system from rejecting the newly transplant-ed organ. The drug also suppresses some of the cells that play a role in the inflammation associated with rheumatoid arthritis.

Cyclosporine isn't prescribed often, but it may be an option for those who don't respond to the more widely used DMARDs, such as methotrexate. It's more effective in combination with other DMARDs than by itself.

Your dosage — between 100 and 400 mg a day in two doses — is determined by your weight. It's important that you take the medication at the same time each day, either with a meal or between meals. The dose is often monitored and adjusted by its level in your blood.

Although cyclosporine doesn't cause problems with the bone marrow — unlike other immunosuppressants and DMARDs such as gold — it can cause the following side effects:

- Kidney damage
- Muscle tremors
- High blood pressure
- Excessive hair growth
- Excessive growth of the gums

This medication can also make you more susceptible to infec-tions and certain cancers. Because of the potential for cyclosporine to cause kidney damage, it's important to have your blood tested. How often you need testing depends on factors such as your response to the medication and whether you have pre-existing heart or kidney problems.

Tell your doctor if you have liver or kidney disease, an infec-tion, or high blood pressure. Don't take this drug with grapefruit, grapefruit juice or St. John's wort, which can affect the drug's absorption.

Cyclophosphamide. Your doctor will turn to cyclophosphamide (Cytoxan) only in very serious situations, such as if your rheuma-toid arthritis extends to other tissues, especially if it inflames your blood vessels. Cyclophosphamide is a drug known as an alkylating agent. These medications are approved for the treatment of cancer, although they are sometimes used to treat rheumatoid arthritis, lupus, scleroderma and other rheumatic diseases.

> **Drug absorption**
>
> The absorption of a medication into your system can be modi-
> fied in different ways.
>
> Taking a drug with food or an antacid can slow or prevent
> the absorption of a drug while protecting your stomach from
> the drug's potentially harsh effects. In fact, some arthritis med-
> ications, such as corticosteroids, are prescribed to be taken with
> food. NSAIDs should be taken with food, liquid or an antacid.
> Others, such as some DMARDs, including minocycline, are pre-
> scribed to be taken on an empty stomach.
>
> The absorption of a medication can also be delayed by taking
> tablets that have an enteric coating. This coating prevents
> absorption until the medication has arrived in the small intes-
> tine, preventing stomach irritation and other problems.

This extremely potent medication kills cells by damaging their
genetic information. In particular, it kills lymphocytes that are part
of an autoimmune disease. Unfortunately, the drug can't tell the
difference between cells that are part of the disease process and
cells that are performing normal functions.

Side effects include:

- Low blood cell counts
- Increased infections
- Bleeding in the bladder, causing blood in urine
- Darkening of skin and fingernails
- Hair loss
- Increased risk of certain cancers, if taken for a long period

Given the potential for serious side effects, your doctor will
want to monitor you very closely while you're taking the drug.
You'll have to have blood tests at regular intervals — every two or
three weeks. You should notify your doctor if you have any problems with bleeding, bruising or fatigue.

You'll take this medication in tablet form with your breakfast.
When you're using the drug, be sure to drink plenty of fluids. Take
care to empty your bladder before going to bed. These steps can
help protect your bladder from possible damage.

If you have an active infection, high blood pressure, or liver or kidney disease, notify your doctor. These conditions may affect your ability to take this medication.

Leflunomide. Leflunomide (Arava) is an immunosuppressant that reduces pain, stiffness, inflammation and swelling. It also may slow or halt joint damage associated with rheumatoid arthritis. People taking the medication generally notice an improvement in symptoms within one to three months.

Similar to other immunosuppressants, leflunomide inhibits certain substances — in this case, a type of enzyme — produced by your immune system. Leflunomide may cause a range of side effects, including abdominal pain, diarrhea, back pain, bronchitis, cough, headache and indigestion. Serious side effects may include liver damage and a reduced ability to fight off infection.

Your doctor will test your liver function before you begin taking the medication and will conduct monthly tests from then on. If you have a liver condition, you may not be able to take leflunomide. If you develop liver problems while taking the drug, your dose will have to be lowered or stopped.

Don't take leflunomide if you're pregnant, breast-feeding or hoping to become pregnant. It can harm the developing fetus and may cause serious side effects in nursing infants. Because of the medication's long half-life, it can take many months to completely eliminate it from your system. If needed, elimination of the drug can be sped up by using cholestyramine, prescribed by your doctor.

Mycophenolate. Mycophenolate (Cellcept) is used to suppress the immune system in people who have received organ transplants. It's called a "prodrug" because after it's given, the body changes it into its active form (mycophenoloic acid). The active drug blocks purine formation which is an essential substance for lymphocyte function. Lymphocytes play a key role in the immune response.

Its use in treating rheumatoid arthritis, systemic erythematosus and other rheumatic diseases has more recently been explored with promising results. Side effects include occasional nausea, vomiting, diarrhea, low white blood cell count and elevated liver enzymes.

Biologic agents

Biologic agents, also called biologic response modifiers (BRMs), are a fairly new class of medications. They interfere with the development or action of cytokines, substances that contribute to arthritis. In response to infection or what it perceives as an invader, your immune system produces cytokines, proteins that influence and mobilize other cells to fight the invader, leading to inflammation.

Biologic drugs differ from conventional drugs because they're derived from living sources, such as cell cultures, while conventional drugs are chemically synthesized.

Biologic agents are among the most effective drugs for improving symptoms, increasing function and slowing progress of rheumatoid arthritis. Two-thirds of people with the disease respond favorably to a biologic agent. These drugs may work for people who have had little success with other medications.

Six biologic agents have received FDA approval:
- Adalimumab (Humira)
- Infliximab (Remicade)
- Etanercept (Enbrel)
- Anakinra (Kineret)
- Abatacept (Orencia)
- Rituximab (Rituxan)

While other immunosuppressant medications affect a larger part of your immune system, the biologic treatments target smaller, specific components of the inflammatory process. Adalimumab, etanercept and infliximab work by blocking a specific cytokine called tumor necrosis factor-alpha (TNF-alpha). Anakinra, works by blocking a cytokine called interleukin-1 (IL-1). Abatacept is a T cell inhibitor and rituximab reduces B cells that have a role in inflammation.

While all three TNF-blocking agents inhibit the action of TNF-alpha, they do it in different ways. Infliximab, adalimumab and rituximab are monoclonal antibodies — proteins produced in the laboratory that capture and remove TNF from the body before it can set off an immune reaction. Etanercept is a soluble cytokine receptor. Etanercept is similar in structure to protein molecules called receptors on the surface of cells that bind, or allow in, TNF. Etanercept competes with these receptors to keep them from bind-ing to TNF. Anakinra interferes with the ability of interleukin-1 to bind with receptor molecules, thus blocking the immune response.

Biologic agents are often used along with DMARDs such as methotrexate. Some biologic agents are also approved for the treatment of other inflammatory diseases. For example, adalimumab is approved as a treatment for psoriatic arthritis. Because these medications are very costly, your doctor might use them only if you haven't responded well to standard DMARDs and other less expensive drugs.

The choice of which biologic medication to use isn't clear-cut. Since the different agents haven't been tested against each other in clinical trials, doctors don't know if one works better than the others for rheumatoid arthritis and other conditions. When choosing a medication, you and your doctor will consider your medical history and any other medical conditions you have, how often you'll take the drug, your preferred way of taking it (injection or infusion), whether you're also taking other medications and which drugs your insurance plan covers.

Adalimumab. Adalimumab (Humira) is the newest TNF-alpha inhibitor. It's approved for first-line treatment of moderate to severe rheumatoid arthritis and for psoriatic arthritis. Like infliximab, adalimumab is a monoclonal antibody, a protein produced in the laboratory from human proteins. It blocks TNF-alpha by neutralizing its biologic activity, reducing the inflammatory process from the start.

Your doctor might prescribe adalimumab alone or in combination with other medications, such as methotrexate. You inject adalimumab under the skin on your thigh, stomach or upper arm every two weeks or weekly, depending on your prescription. The medication comes in a prefilled, premeasured syringe.

The most common side effect is a mild reaction at the injection site, such as redness, pain, itching, swelling or bruising. Other side effects include upper respiratory (sinus) infections, headaches and nausea. Serious side effects are rare but may include development of a serious infection (such as tuberculosis), a nervous system disorder or certain kinds of cancer, such as lymphoma. Some people who take this drug get lupus-like symptoms that go away when they stop taking the medication.

In rare instances, adalimumab may cause a severe allergic reaction or a blood disorder called cytopenia. Discontinue use and see your doctor if you have an allergic reaction (such as difficulty breathing, hives and itching, or a weak or rapid pulse), if you have a serious or recurrent infection (such as pneumonia), or if you have a persistent fever, bruising, bleeding or paleness.

People with congestive heart failure shouldn't take adalimumab. Also let your doctor know if you have an active infection or a nervous system disorder, such as multiple sclerosis.

Infliximab. Infliximab (Remicade) works in a similar way as adalimumab to block the action of TNF-alpha. For the majority of people, infliximab will ease signs and symptoms of rheumatoid arthritis. Studies show that even if you notice little improvement in symptoms when taking infliximab, it still protects against joint damage.

Like the other biologic agents, infliximab is more costly and complicated to administer and therefore is generally prescribed when other medications haven't been effective. Infliximab is given with methotrexate to enhance its effectiveness and reduce side effects.

Infliximab is given by intravenous (IV) infusion in a doctor's office, clinic or hospital. The process involves inserting a tiny tube (catheter) into your arm. The drug is administered through the catheter over a two-hour period. Additional doses are given at two weeks and six weeks. Maintenance doses are usually administered every eight weeks.

Side effects of the medication may include respiratory problems, sore throat, abdominal pain, rash, fever, headache, nausea, diarrhea and worsening of congestive heart failure. You may have a reaction to the infusion during or shortly after it. This may include chest pain, change in blood pressure, difficulty breathing and hives. Your doctor may treat you in advance with a pain reliever, antihistamine or steroid medication to prevent such a reaction.

Like adalimumab and etanercept, infliximab also weakens your immune system response. Because of the increased risk of infections such as tuberculosis, you should have a negative TB test before beginning treatment with infliximab.

Filtering out harmful substances

A unique method for treating rheumatoid arthritis involves a blood-filtering device. The technique — called selective extra-corporeal immunoadsorption column (Prosorba column) — works somewhat like kidney dialysis.

Blood is drawn from a vein in your arm and then pumped through a cell separator (apheresis machine). This machine separates the liquid part of your blood (plasma) from blood cells. The plasma then passes through the Prosorba column, a plastic cylinder about the size of a coffee mug. The cylinder contains a sand-like substance coated with a special material called protein A. Protein A is thought to bind to certain substances (immune complexes and antigens involved in the inflammatory process), removing the substances from your blood. The filtered plasma is reunited with your blood cells and returned to your body through a vein in your other arm. The procedure takes about two hours.

A few people have developed symptoms of autoimmune disorders, such as lupus or multiple sclerosis, while taking infliximab. In addition, studies have shown an increased risk of lymphoma and abnormal cell growth among people taking infliximab.

If you have another health condition or are taking medications that can weaken your immune system, you may not be a candidate for infliximab. And you shouldn't take this medication if you have congestive heart failure.

Etanercept. Etanercept (Enbrel) is used to treat moderate to severe rheumatoid arthritis, as well as psoriatic arthritis, juvenile rheumatoid arthritis and ankylosing spondylitis. The drug mimics the action of TNF-alpha receptors naturally found in your body, "soaking up" excess TNF-alpha, which helps to reduce the inflammation.

Etanercept has been shown to provide significant symptom relief. The drug can be taken along with other medications commonly used to treat rheumatoid arthritis, including methotrexate, corticosteroids and pain relievers.

Because the drug is more costly and more complicated to take than some other arthritis medications, etanercept is generally

The number of treatments you receive is based on your condition. One treatment a week for 12 weeks is typical. Not everyone responds to the treatment, but in clinical studies, many participants noticed at least some improvement in symptoms. It often takes one to three months before benefits of this therapy are noticeable. The most common side effects are flu-like conditions and a short-term flare in joint pain and swelling for a couple of days after treatment.

This technique is generally reserved for people with severe rheumatoid arthritis who haven't improved after treatment with DMARDs and biologic agents. Because the filtering process can lower your blood pressure, you may not be a candidate for this therapy if you have a heart condition or are taking medication for high blood pressure.

prescribed when traditional medications have proved inadequate. Etanercept is given twice a week by injection under the skin of your thigh, abdomen or upper arm. You may be able to take a larger dose once a week instead. You can inject the medication yourself at home or receive the injections at your doctor's office.

Side effects of the medication may include abdominal pain, fever, reduced white blood cell count, dizziness, headache, indigestion, respiratory problems and injection site reactions, such as rash and itching. Serious, even fatal, infections may occur, especially in people whose immune systems are already weakened. People taking this drug should avoid exposure to infection, including fungal infections and tuberculosis.

If you're taking medications that can weaken your immune system, you may not be a candidate for etanercept. In addition, because it may worsen congestive heart failure, people with this disorder shouldn't take etanercept.

This medication has been associated in rare circumstances with severe, even fatal, blood disorders. Tell your doctor if you notice persistent bruising, bleeding or paleness.

Biologic medications and infections

Tumor necrosis factor-alpha (TNF-alpha) is a key player in your immune system's response to infection by bacteria, viruses and other invaders. When a foreign invader is discovered, white blood cells in your body synthesize increased amounts of TNF-alpha. The TNF-alpha mobilizes white blood cells to the area to engage in battle and destroy the invaders. This temporarily causes inflammation.

Normally, after the infection is cleared up, your body stops making excess TNF-alpha. But if you have rheumatoid arthritis, your body continues to make excess TNF-alpha. As it builds up, more and more white blood cells travel to the affected area. This causes the inflammation, pain and tissue damage of arthritis. The biologic medications adalimumab, infliximab and etanercept block the action of TNF-alpha, thereby reducing inflammation.

By decreasing the action of TNF-alpha, however, these biologic agents also limit your body's ability to fight infections. People taking these drugs have reported a number of infections ranging from sinus infections to tuberculosis. Most of the people who developed a serious infection while taking a biologic agent were also taking other medications that suppress the immune system, such as methotrexate or a corticosteroid.

Anakinra. Anakinra (Kineret) works by inhibiting interleukin-1 (IL-1), another protein that promotes inflammation. Like other biologic agents, anakinra is effective in reducing the pain and swelling of rheumatoid arthritis. It also slows the progression of joint damage.

Also like those other agents, anakinra is expensive and used mainly for people who aren't responding to conventional treatment. Because of the cost and the need for daily injections, anakinra tends to be used only if another biologic agent hasn't worked.

The daily dose is given by self-administered injection under the skin of your thigh, upper arm or abdomen. You may use prefilled syringes and an automatic injection device. Benefits of anakinra

The risk of serious infection also increases if you take a TNF-alpha inhibitor along with the interleukin-1 antagonist anakinra. You shouldn't take both types of biologic agents at the same time.

Before prescribing any biologic agent, including anakinra, your doctor will ask you about any current or recurring infections you may have. Your doctor will also want to test you for tuberculosis, as well as fungal infections such as histoplasmosis and coccidioidomycosis (valley fever), since these may worsen if you're being treated with a TNF-alpha inhibitor.

If you do develop an infection while taking any biologic agent, you may have to stop the treatment until your infection has been successfully treated.

Another job of TNF-alpha is to help the immune system protect the body from abnormal growths, such as cancerous (malignant) tumors. TNF-alpha plays a role in destroying some types of tumor cells. It's not clear whether TNF-alpha inhibitors can cause cancers such as lymphoma. People with rheumatoid arthritis have an increased risk of lymphoma even if they're not being treated with TNF-alpha inhibitors. So far research hasn't shown a clear link between these drugs and an increased risk of cancer, but long-term studies are needed.

may be evident in the first week of treatment, but the maximum results may not be felt for a month or longer.

Side effects of anakinra include rash and itching at the injection site, which can be treated with a mild steroid cream. Other infrequent side effects include temporary reduction in white blood cell count, headache and an increase in upper respiratory infections. Serious infections, such as pneumonia, occur in a small percentage of people taking this medication.

Abatacept. Abatacept (Orencia) is a selective costimulation modulator that inhibits T cell activation. It received FDA approval in late 2005. T cells, which play a role in inflammation, require two signals to turn them on. Abatacept interferes with one of those signals and renders T cells less active. Abatacept is used to reduce the signs and symptoms of moderate to severe rheumatoid arthritis in people who have not been helped by other medications. Specifically, abatacept has been shown to reduce inflammation, slow damage to joints and improve physical function. In one study, 68 percent of people with rheumatoid arthritis who took abatacept showed signs of improvement after six months.

Because it interferes with the immune response system, abatacept may lower your ability to fight infection. Side effects include headache, upper respiratory infection, sore throat and nausea. Abatacept should not be taken with TNF blockers, and caution is advised if you have chronic obstructive pulmonary disease.

Rituximab. Rituximab (Rituxan) is a genetically engineered protein that binds to B cells, causing them to self-destruct. B cells have an important role in the development of rheumatoid arthritis. Rituximab was approved for treatment of rheumatoid arthritis in early 2006. For more on rituximab, see pages 136 and 201.

Penicillamine

Penicillamine (Cuprimine, Depen Titratabs) is approved for the treatment of rheumatoid arthritis, but it's generally no longer used. The medication can reduce inflammation, but side effects can be severe.

Topical pain relievers

Topical pain relievers are creams, lotions, gels or sprays that you put on your skin. Available as OTC products, they can temporarily ease some types of arthritis pain.

Topical pain relievers work in different ways. Some (ArthriCare, Eucalyptamint, Icy Hot, Therapeutic Mineral Ice) contain skin irritants such as menthol, oil of wintergreen or eucalyptus oil, which produce a sensation of cold or heat that distracts from the arthritis pain. Other topical agents contain salicylates, the same ingredients that give aspirin its pain-relieving quality. In addition to relieving pain, products with salicylates (BenGay, Aspercreme, Flexall, Mobisyl, Sportscreme) may reduce inflammation in muscles and joints by being absorbed through the skin.

Capsaicin (Capzasin-P, Zostrix, Zostrix HP) is a cream made from the seeds of hot chili peppers. It's most effective for arthritic joints close to your skin surface, such as your fingers, knees and elbows. Capsaicin works by depleting your nerve cells of a chemical called substance P, which is important for sending pain messages. You rub the medication on your skin three or four times a day. You may feel an initial burning or stinging sensation, but this usually goes away with repeated applications. It may take a week or two before you begin to feel pain relief.

When using topical pain relievers, be careful not to rub or touch your eyes until you've washed your hands thoroughly. Don't use these pain relievers on broken or irritated skin or in combination with a heating pad or bandage. If you're allergic to aspirin or are taking an anticoagulant blood thinner, check with your doctor before using topical medications that contain salicylates.

Antidepressant drugs

Depression is common among people with chronic pain. In studies of people with chronic diseases, about one in three people report feelings of depression. Some studies suggest that more than half of people with rheumatoid arthritis experience symptoms of depression.

If you've experienced depression along with arthritis, your doctor may prescribe an antidepressant drug. These prescription medications can help treat the depression and insomnia that often accompany chronic pain.

Even if you don't have depression, antidepressants can help relieve pain. Depression adversely influences the perception of pain and its intensity. Several studies have shown that in people diagnosed with both arthritis and depression, treating the depression can improve symptoms of arthritis. Prescribed in low doses and taken at bedtime, antidepressants may also help you sleep better.

Because these drugs cause some side effects and vary in effectiveness from one person to another, your doctor may have you try different drugs until you find one that works best for you.

Tricyclic antidepressants are most often prescribed for people with arthritis. These include the following:

- Amitriptyline
- Desipramine (Norpramin)
- Imipramine (Tofranil, Tofranil-PM)
- Nortriptyline (Aventyl, Pamelor)

If tricyclic antidepressants prove ineffective, your doctor may prescribe other antidepressants, such as:

- Sertraline (Zoloft)
- Trazodone (Desyrel)

Antidepressants aren't addictive, so you can use them for a long time. Possible side effects include drowsiness, constipation, difficulty with urination, weight gain, blurred vision and dry mouth. If you're experiencing dry mouth from taking an antidepressant, ask your doctor about switching to a different drug.

Muscle relaxants

Muscle relaxants such as cyclobenzaprine (Flexeril) or carisoprodol (Soma) relax the muscles. They're often used to relieve pain triggered by muscle spasms associated with injury of muscles, bones and joints. Muscle relaxants may help people with fibromyalgia. However, with arthritis, they haven't proved useful.

Benzodiazepines

Even in low doses, tranquilizers such as diazepam (Valium), alprazolam (Xanax) and chlordiazepoxide (Librium) can cause dependency when taken over a period of time. In addition, these depressant drugs can be extremely dangerous when mixed with alcohol. Because tranquilizers aren't effective for treating arthritis and may actually cause depression, it's best not to take them for arthritis symptoms.

Hyaluronic acid derivatives

Hyaluronic acid, or hyaluronate, is a natural substance found in normal joint fluid. It helps form a "microlayer" of lubrication between the bones of joints as they move. If you have osteoarthritis, the hyaluronic acid molecules are altered and their lubricating effect is reduced. This could result in more rapid wearing down of the joints. For people with osteoarthritis in one or both knees, injecting a compound containing hyaluronic acid into a diseased knee joint is thought to restore more normal joint lubrication. Injecting hyaluronic acid derivatives into joints can improve mobility and reduce pain, although there's no evidence that the injections slow progression of the disease.

Hyaluronic acid injections may be recommended for people with osteoarthritis who don't get relief from other medications, exercise or physical therapy. Several forms of hyaluronic acid are available, sold under the brand names Hyalgan, Euflexxa, Orthovisc, Supartz and Synvisc.

Hyaluronic acid is given in a series of three to five injections. A local anesthetic is injected first to ease discomfort from the medication, which must be administered with a large-gauge needle.

Relief may last up to six months or longer. If the first series of shots provides pain relief, a second round may be given, perhaps with longer-lasting effects.

The most common side effects are pain, swelling or a rash at the injection site. Other side effects may include headache, nausea, abdominal pain or other gastrointestinal complaints, and muscle pain.

Arthritis medications guide

Pain reducers (analgesics)

Generic names	Brand names
Acetaminophen	Tylenol,* others

- **Possible side effects:** High blood pressure.
- **Reminders and cautions:** High doses of acetaminophen may cause liver damage. Using this drug with alcohol can also cause liver damage. Avoid using this medication if you consume more than three alcoholic drinks a day.

Available without a prescription.

Codeine	

- **Possible side effects:** Constipation, lightheadedness, dizziness, nausea, sedation, shortness of breath and mood changes.
- **Reminders and cautions:** Tell your doctor if you're constipated. Also, be aware that this narcotic can be addictive.

Hydrocodone with acetaminophen	Hydrocet, Lorcet, Lortab, Vicodin

- **Possible side effects:** Lightheadedness, dizziness, sedation, nausea, vomiting and mood changes.
- **Reminders and cautions:** Tell your doctor if you're constipated. Also, be aware that this narcotic can be addictive.

Hydrocodone with ibuprofen   Vicoprofen

- **Possible side effects:** Anxiety, insomnia, nervousness, tingling, sweating, diarrhea, gas, upset stomach, stomach cramps, dry mouth and swelling.
- **Reminders and cautions:** Use of this drug can lead to dependency. Notify your doctor if you're allergic to aspirin or are taking heparin, naltrexone or sodium oxybate. Also see the cautions listed for NSAIDs on page 129.

Meperidine   Demerol

- **Possible side effects:** Constipation, vomiting, nausea, lightheadedness, dizziness, sedation and sweating.
- **Reminders and cautions:** Use of this drug can lead to dependency. Notify your doctor if you have severe kidney or liver problems, hypothyroidism, Addison's disease, head injury, irregular heartbeat, or if you have ever had convulsions.

Morphine sulfate   Avinza, MSIR, MS Contin, Oramorph SR

- **Possible side effects:** Constipation, drowsiness and nausea.
- **Reminders and cautions:** Use of this drug can lead to dependency. Notify your doctor if you have liver problems or use central nervous system depressants such as antihistamines or muscle relaxants.

Oxycodone   OxyContin, OxyFAST, OxyIR, Roxicodone

- **Possible side effects:** Vomiting, nausea, lightheadedness, dizziness, headache, dry mouth, sweating, itching, shortness of breath and sedation.
- **Reminders and cautions:** Tell your doctor if you have a head injury, stomach problems, kidney, liver or thyroid disease, Addison's disease, an enlarged prostate, or drug or alcohol abuse problems. Don't take this drug with alcohol. Use of this drug may lead to dependency.

ARTHRITIS MEDICATIONS GUIDE

Oxycodone with acetaminophen	Endocet, Percocet, Roxicet, Tylox

- **Possible side effects:** Vomiting, nausea, lightheadedness, dizziness, headache, dry mouth, sweating, itching, shortness of breath and sedation.
- **Reminders and cautions:** Tell your doctor if you have a head injury, stomach problems, kidney, liver or thyroid disease, Addison's disease, an enlarged prostate, or drug or alcohol abuse problems. Don't take this drug with alcohol. Use of this drug may lead to dependency.

Oxycodone with aspirin	Endodan, Percodan

- **Possible side effects:** Drowsiness, dizziness, lightheadedness, upset stomach, nausea and vomiting.
- **Reminders and cautions:** Avoid this medication if you're allergic to aspirin, if you're pregnant or are planning to become pregnant, if you regularly consume alcoholic beverages, or if you have ulcers, stomach problems, a blood clotting disorder, kidney or liver problems or an underactive thyroid. Use of this drug may lead to dependency.

Propoxyphene	Darvon, Darvon-N

- **Possible side effects:** Vomiting, nausea, lightheadedness, dizziness, drowsiness and sedation.
- **Reminders and cautions:** Tell your doctor if you have ever experienced serious depression or are using antidepressants or tranquilizers, if you have a kidney or liver problem, or if you are pregnant or plan to become pregnant.

Propoxyphene with acetaminophen Darvocet-N

- **Possible side effects:** Vomiting, nausea, lightheadedness, dizziness, drowsiness and sedation.
- **Reminders and cautions:** Tell your doctor if you have ever experienced serious depression or are using antidepressants or tranquilizers, if you have a kidney or liver problem, or if you are pregnant or plan to become pregnant.

Tramadol   Ultram

- **Possible side effects:** Upset stomach, nausea, constipation, drowsiness, increased sweating and occasional dizziness.
- **Reminders and cautions:** Tell your doctor of any medications you are taking, because this drug can be involved in drug interactions and can cause seizures, especially in people taking other medications.

Tramadol with acetaminophen   Ultracet

- **Possible side effects:** Upset stomach, nausea, constipation, drowsiness, increased sweating and occasional dizziness
- **Reminders and cautions:** Tell your doctor of any medications you're taking, because this drug can be involved in drug interactions and can cause seizures, especially in people taking other medications.

ARTHRITIS MEDICATIONS GUIDE

NSAIDs

Generic names	Brand names
Aspirin	Anacin,* Ascriptin,* Aspergum,* Bayer,* Bufferin,* Ecotrin,* Halfprin 81,* Norwich,* St. Joseph,* ZORprin*
Choline magnesium trisalicylate	
Diclofenac	Cataflam, Voltaren, Voltaren-XR
Diclofenac and misoprostol	Arthrotec
Diflunisal	Dolobid
Etodolac	Lodine, Lodine XL
Fenoprofen calcium	
Flurbiprofen	Ansaid
Ibuprofen	Advil,* Motrin IB,* Midol Cramps & Body Aches
Indomethacin	Indocin, Indocin SR
Ketoprofen	Orudis,* Oruvail
Magnesium salicylate	Doan's*
Meclofenamate sodium	Meclomen
Mefenamic acid	Ponstel
Meloxicam	Mobic
Nabumetone	Relafen
Naproxen	Naprelan, Naprosyn
Naproxen with lansoprazole	Prevacid NapraPAC
Naproxen sodium	Aleve,* Anaprox, Anaprox DS
Oxaprozin	Daypro
Piroxicam	Feldene
Salsalate	Amigesic, Artha-G, Mono-Gesic, Salflex*
Sulindac	Clinoril
Tolmetin	Tolectin, Tolectin DS

- **Possible side effects:** Mild headache, lightheadedness, drowsiness, dizziness, heartburn, stomach irritation, gastric ulcers and bleeding, nausea or vomiting, decreased kidney function, ringing in the ears, swelling of the feet, fluid retention, mouth sores, skin rashes and more-serious skin reactions. Taking non-aspirin NSAIDs may increase risk of high blood pressure and cardiovascular problems such as heart attack and stroke.

- **Reminders and cautions:** Tell your doctor if you are allergic to aspirin or similar medications, have kidney, liver or heart disease, have high blood pressure, stomach ulcers or asthma, or use blood thinners. Avoid these drugs if you've had recent coronary bypass surgery, a stroke or transient ischemic attacks (TIAs). Some NSAIDs increase your sensitivity to sunlight — limit your exposure by staying out of direct sunlight during the middle of the day, wearing protective clothing and using sunscreen.

*Available without a prescription.

COX-2 inhibitors

Generic name	Brand name
Celecoxib	Celebrex

- **Possible side effects:** Increased risk of cardiovascular problems including heart attack and stroke, respiratory infection or inflammation, headache, dizziness, diarrhea, nausea, heartburn, stomach pain, high blood pressure, swelling of the legs and feet, back pain, urinary tract infection, allergic reaction, decreased kidney function, gastrointestinal ulceration and bleeding and elevated liver enzymes.
- **Reminders and cautions:** Tell your doctor if you are allergic to aspirin or similar medications, have kidney, liver or heart disease, have high blood pressure, peptic ulcers or asthma, or use blood thinners. Avoid this drug if you've had coronary bypass surgery, a stroke or transient ischemic attacks (TIAs).

Corticosteroids

Generic names	Brand names
Betamethasone	Celestone, Celestone Soluspan
Cortisone acetate	
Dexamethasone	Decadron
Hydrocortisone	Cortef, Hydrocortone
Methylprednisolone	Medrol
Prednisolone	Prelone
Prednisone	
Triamcinolone	Aristocort, Kenalog

- **Possible side effects:** Weight gain, mood swings, nervousness, insomnia, indigestion, muscle weakness, bruising, and thin skin. People taking moderate or high doses may have an increased blood sugar level, high blood pressure, elevated blood fats, hardening of arteries, stomach ulcers or irritation (usually when NSAIDs are also being taken), osteoporosis, risk of infection, purple or red stretch marks.

- **Reminders and cautions:** Dependency can develop because the adrenal glands stop making cortisol, resulting in a potentially dangerous condition called adrenal crisis. If you use corticosteroids for a long time, wear a medical alert bracelet or necklace. Drug interactions are possible, so be sure to inform your doctor of other medications you take. Tell your doctor if you have a fungal infection, history of tuberculosis, underactive thyroid, diabetes, stomach ulcer, high blood pressure or osteoporosis.

DMARDs

Generic names	Brand names
Hydroxychloroquine	Plaquenil

- **Possible side effects:** Blurred vision, diarrhea, headache, itching, loss of appetite and rashes. Rare side effects include damage to the eyes, upset stomach and muscle weakness.
- **Reminders and cautions:** When using this drug, you may want to wear sunglasses and a broad-brimmed hat in the sun. Have your eyes checked every six to 12 months.

Gold compounds	Myochrysine, Ridaura

- **Possible side effects:** Diarrhea, metallic taste in mouth, mouth sores, gum and tongue irritation or soreness, kidney damage, bone marrow damage, itching and skin rashes. With injectable gold, joint pain may occur for one or two days after receiving an injection.
- **Reminders and cautions:** Tell your doctor if you have kidney or liver disease, a blood cell abnormality or inflammatory bowel disease or have had a negative reaction to this drug in the past. Gold compounds can cause sun sensitivity, so limit your exposure to the sun by staying out of direct sunlight during the middle of the day, wearing protective clothing and using sunscreen.

Sulfasalazine	Azulfidine, Azulfidine EN-Tabs

- **Possible side effects:** Nausea, stomach distress, loss of appetite, vomiting, headache, itching or rash, fever, joint aching, increased sun sensitivity and anemia.
- **Reminders and cautions:** Tell your doctor if you have a sensitivity to sulfa drugs or aspirin, have liver, kidney or blood disease, or have bronchial asthma. Be sure to drink plenty of fluids while using this drug.

Minocycline	Minocin, Dynacin

- **Possible side effects:** Liver damage, nausea, stomach cramps, darkening of the skin, rash, dizziness, headache, vaginal infections, anemia, appetite loss and diarrhea.
- **Reminders and cautions:** This drug is a tetracycline antibiotic. It isn't FDA-approved for arthritis but is used off label for rheumatoid arthritis. Consult your doctor before taking this drug with antacids, blood thinners, preparations with iron, oral contraceptives or penicillin. If you are pregnant or plan to become pregnant, inform your doctor before taking this drug.

Immunosuppressants

Generic names	Brand names
Azathioprine	Imuran

- **Possible side effects:** Decreased ability to fight infection, gastrointestinal distress, easy bleeding and bruising, fatigue, loss of appetite, fevers and chills.
- **Reminders and cautions:** Avoid taking this drug if you have liver or kidney disease. Don't take with the gout drug allopurinol. Azathioprine may be associated with the development of certain cancers.

Mycophenolate	Cellcept

- **Possible side effects:** Nausea, vomiting, low blood cell counts and elevated liver enzymes.
- **Reminders and cautions:** Don't take with azathioprine. Rare risk of malignancy reported.

Cyclophosphamide	Cytoxan

- **Possible side effects:** Low blood cell counts, increased infections, blood in urine, darkening of skin and fingernails, hair loss, increased risk of certain cancers if taken for a long period, and damage to bone marrow, stomach or bowels.
- **Reminders and cautions:** Tell your doctor if you have an active infection or liver or kidney disease. This drug is an anti-cancer agent that's not FDA-approved for arthritis but is used off label in treating rheumatoid arthritis.

Cyclosporine	Gengraf, Neoral

- **Possible side effects:** Kidney damage or failure, headache, high blood pressure, muscle tremors, loss of appetite, nausea, excessive hair growth and excessive growth of the gums. Use of this drug may make you more susceptible to infections and certain cancers.
- **Reminders and cautions:** Tell your doctor if you are pregnant or plan to become pregnant or if you have kidney or liver disease, high blood pressure or an infection. Interactions can occur with many other drugs when taking cyclosporine. Avoid having immunizations or vaccinations while taking this drug. Don't take it with grapefruit, grapefruit juice or St. John's wort.

Leflunomide	Arava

- **Possible side effects:** Diarrhea, headache, dizziness, temporary loss of hair, rash, stomach pain, sneezing, sore throat, high blood pressure and liver problems.
- **Reminders and cautions:** Tell your doctor if you have an infection, liver or kidney disease, or cancer. Men and women who are trying to conceive shouldn't take this drug.

ARTHRITIS MEDICATIONS GUIDE

Methotrexate	Rheumatrex, Trexall

- **Possible side effects:** Nausea or stomach pain, diarrhea, loss of appetite, headache, chills, fever, increased sun sensitivity, itching, hair loss, mouth ulcers or sores, rashes, easy bruising or bleeding, liver problems, skin rashes and fatigue. This drug may be associated with an increased risk of lymphoma.
- **Reminders and cautions:** Tell your doctor if you are pregnant, are breast-feeding, have kidney or liver disease, have allergies to medications, are exposed to people with infections, have been treated with X-rays or cancer drugs, or use alcohol. Alert your doctor immediately if you have a dry cough, fever or difficulty breathing.

Biologic agents

Generic names	Brand names
Abatacept	Orencia

- **Possible side effects:** Headache, upper respiratory infections, sore throat, nausea, sinusitis, pneumonia, influenza, cellulitis, bronchitis, diverticulitis, urinary tract infection and acute pyelonephritis.
- **Reminders and cautions:** Tell your doctor if you have a weakened immune system or history of recurring infection, you develop an allergic reaction or infection while taking the medication, or you are pregnant or are planning to become pregnant in the near future. Caution is advised if you take this drug and have chronic obstructive pulmonary disease (COPD). This drug should not be taken with tumor necrosis factor inhibitors. Vaccination with live vaccine should be avoided while taking this drug, and within three months of its discontinuation.

Adalimumab	Humira

- **Possible side effects:** Injection site reactions (rash, itching, hives), upper respiratory infections, abdominal pain, nausea, sinus and nasal inflammation, headache, urinary tract infection, rash, back pain, elevated blood fats and high blood pressure.
- **Reminders and cautions:** Tell your doctor if you have a weakened immune system or history of recurring infection, you develop an allergic reaction or infection while taking the medication, you are pregnant or breast-feeding, or you plan to become pregnant in the near future. Don't take this drug if you have congestive heart failure. This drug shouldn't be taken in combination with anakinra.

Anakinra	Kineret

- **Possible side effects:** Injection site reactions (rash, itching, hives), flu-like symptoms, including cough, runny nose and headache, and lowered white blood cell count.
- **Reminders and cautions:** Tell your doctor if you have a weakened immune system or history of recurring infection or asthma, you develop an allergic reaction or infection while taking the medication, you are pregnant or breast-feeding, or you plan to become pregnant in the near future. This drug shouldn't be taken in combination with adalimumab.

Etanercept	Enbrel

- **Possible side effects:** Injection site reactions (rash, itching, hives), abdominal pain, cough, dizziness, headache, indigestion, infection, rash, nausea, respiratory problems, sinus and nasal inflammation, sore throat, chest pain or heart attack, high or low blood pressure, stomach and intestinal bleeding, and lowered white blood cell count. Rarely, use of this drug has been associated with the development of lupus and multiple sclerosis.

ARTHRITIS MEDICATIONS GUIDE

- **Reminders and cautions:** Tell your doctor if you have a weakened immune system or history of recurring infection, you develop an allergic reaction or infection while taking the medication, you are pregnant or breast-feeding, or you plan to become pregnant in the near future. Don't take this drug if you have congestive heart failure.

Infliximab	Remicade

- **Possible side effects:** Infusion site reaction (hives), respiratory problems, headache, fever, diarrhea, indigestion, infection, cough, difficulty breathing and low blood pressure. May also cause severe liver problems, including liver failure, jaundice and hepatitis. Rarely has been associated with the development of lupus and multiple sclerosis.
- **Reminders and cautions:** Tell your doctor if you have a weakened immune system or history of recurring infection, you have a nervous system disorder such as multiple sclerosis, you develop an allergic reaction or infection while taking the medication, you are pregnant or breast-feeding, or you plan to become pregnant in the near future. Have a tuberculosis skin test before taking this drug. Don't take it if you have congestive heart failure.

Rituximab	Rituxan

- **Possible side effects:** Black, tarry stools, bleeding gums, bloating and swelling, blood in urine and stools, blurred vision, cough or hoarseness, dizziness, dry mouth, fatigue, fever and chills.
- **Reminders and cautions:** Tell your doctor if you are breast-feeding, pregnant or think you're pregnant; if you have heart or lung problems, or hepatitis B.

Chapter 6

Surgical treatments

If joint pain is keeping you on the sidelines and other therapies haven't helped, then a surgical procedure may be one way to a more active, satisfying life. Your doctor may recommend some form of joint operation when other treatments such as medications, physical therapy and weight loss fail to relieve your arthritis symptoms. Surgeons use various procedures to relieve pain, slow or prevent cartilage damage, and restore mobility and stability.

Because joint operations pose some risks, it's a good idea to discuss these issues with your doctor before deciding whether it's the best option for you. The strength of your bones and the ligaments supporting your joints, your age, your weight and your ability to participate in rehabilitation can all affect the outcome of a joint operation. It's also important to understand and accept the limits that such surgery may impose.

Selecting a surgeon

Your personal physician can help you obtain consultation with a surgeon. He or she will usually recommend an orthopedic surgeon who has extensive experience in joint procedures. Orthopedic surgeons perform operations involving joints, muscles and bones.

Board-certified orthopedic surgeons have met training and experience requirements beyond those required for licensure. Some orthopedic surgeons complete additional training and focus their practice on the treatment of specific joints.

It's important to have confidence in the surgeon you choose. An experienced surgeon should be able to answer your questions about the surgical options available to you, the risks and benefits associated with each and what to expect during your recovery.

Given the potential risks and costs associated with surgery, seeking a second opinion before proceeding with an operation may be a sensible option. Either you or your primary physician can initiate the process to get a second opinion. Don't be afraid to bring it up.

Common forms of joint surgery

Many types of surgical procedures are used to treat joints affected by arthritis. Depending on your age and overall health, the form of arthritis you have and your specific joint problems, your surgeon may recommend one or more of the following procedures.

Arthroscopic debridement

Surgeons use this procedure to remove loose fragments of bone, cartilage or synovium that cause joint pain, most often in the knees. During this procedure, the surgeon makes a small incision and inserts an arthroscope. This device is a thin tube through which the surgeon views and suctions out the tissue fragments. In some cases the surgeon may need to insert other surgical instruments through additional small incisions. This procedure is often helpful to people with osteoarthritis.

Synovectomy

The purpose of this procedure is to remove some of the inflamed synovial tissue that lines joints affected by inflammatory arthritis, especially rheumatoid arthritis. Removing this tissue can reduce pain and swelling and delay or possibly prevent the destruction of the cartilage and bone. Although it can provide pain relief, synovectomy is not a cure. The inflammation may recur as the synovium regrows after the operation.

Synovectomy is routinely performed on the fingers, wrists and knees, before significant cartilage erosion or deformity occurs. The procedure is best left to an experienced surgeon. Some specialists also perform synovectomy on the elbow.

Cartilage replacement

In cartilage transplantation, cartilage cells are removed from one of your healthy joints, grown in a laboratory and then inserted into a damaged joint along with a solution that stimulates growth.

Physicians are now using cartilage transplantation to treat only small areas of damaged cartilage. The ability to repair larger areas is likely to be developed in the next five to 10 years. Identifying and producing substances that stimulate healthy cartilage growth (cartilage growth factors) may help advance this technique.

Osteotomy

During this procedure, surgeons cut and reposition bones near a damaged joint to help correct deformities caused by arthritis. These adjustments also help slow cartilage damage by distributing your body weight more evenly across the joint. Osteotomy is sometimes used to correct curvature or bowing in the lower leg bones caused by osteoarthritis.

Resection

Surgeons sometimes remove all or part of a damaged bone when diseased joints make movement painful. Resection is frequently used in the feet to make walking easier and in the wrists and hands to reduce pain.

Joint replacement (arthroplasty)

When osteoarthritis or rheumatoid arthritis severely damages a joint, your doctor may recommend a surgical procedure called arthroplasty (AHR-thro-plas-tee). Arthroplasty literally means "reforming of the joint." The operation may involve smoothing the ends of bones in a joint.

Anatomy of an artificial joint

Artificial joint implants are made of various metals, ceramics or plasticlike materials called polymers. Common polymers used in artificial joints include acrylic, nylon, silicone, polyurethane, polyethylene and polypropylene. At some medical centers, physicians sometimes use computers to custom design an implant and plan the operation. Large inventories of artificial joints enable surgeons to select the implant best suited to your needs.

Traditionally, surgeons have secured joint implants to bones with a bone cement (methylmethacrylate). But this cement can crack after several years, causing the implant to loosen. If loosening occurs, you may need additional operations to reattach or replace the implant. To fix this problem, researchers are exploring new methods of manufacturing and applying the cement.

In some cases, cementless prostheses may improve the durability of implants. These implants have a porous surface into which the bone grows and attaches itself (bone ingrowth). But cementless implants also can loosen.

Over time, both types of artificial joints create debris caused by friction and wear. The shedding of particles can cause irritation that destroys bone and ultimately contributes to loosening. Gradual deterioration of the hip joint can occur in osteoarthritis. Implanting an artificial hip can help to eliminate pain and restore near-normal function.

In replacement arthroplasty, also called total joint replacement, surgeons remove certain parts of the damaged joint and replace them with a high-density plastic or metal alloy device called a prosthesis or implant. Implants are made of several different materials, including polyethylene and various metals. The hip and the knee are the most commonly replaced joints, but implants can also replace shoulder, elbow, finger and other joints.

Joint fusion

Also called arthrodesis (ahr-thro-DEE-sis), joint fusion is used most often to reduce pain and improve stability in the spine, wrist, fingers, ankle and feet. During this procedure surgeons remove a thin layer of tissue from the ends of two bones and bind them together, often using pins, rods or plates. Fresh bone cells then grow and fuse the two bones. Once healed, the fused joint can bear weight, but it has no flexibility. Because it eliminates joint mobility, joint fusion is typically used when total joint replacement isn't possible.

Tendon and ligament adjustments
Surgeons can repair tendon tears to reduce pain, restore function and, in some cases, prevent tendon rupture. Procedures to tighten or loosen tendons and ligaments are sometimes recommended to decrease pain, increase joint mobility or prepare a joint for total joint replacement. Surgeons also perform procedures to relieve pressure on nerves located near damaged joints.

Which joints can surgery help?

Because your joints vary in size, shape and design, surgeons must tailor their treatments to accommodate these differences. This section explains how surgeons use the various surgical procedures to relieve arthritis symptoms in specific joints.

Hand and wrist joints
The ability to grasp a spoon, turn a doorknob or open a can of soda is something you may not take for granted if arthritis affects your hands or wrists. It's no secret that arthritis pain can make these movements difficult, if not nearly impossible.

Like all joint operations, the goal of procedures on the hands and wrists is to improve function and reduce pain. Although some procedures can improve the appearance of joints deformed by arthritis, surgery is rarely recommended for cosmetic reasons alone. However, you may be a candidate for surgery if the appearance of your hands or wrists is having a profoundly detrimental effect on your self-image and social interactions.

Sometimes, rheumatoid arthritis causes tears in the tendons of the hand and wrist, and an operation is performed to repair the

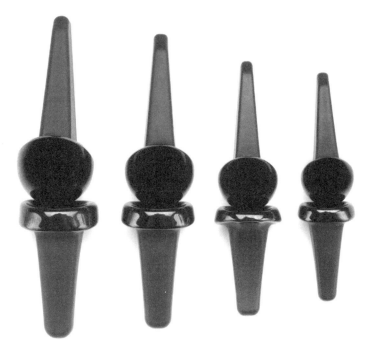

Finger joint implants are designed to replace joints that have degenerated from arthritis and are no longer flexible. The surgeon determines the type and size of implant.

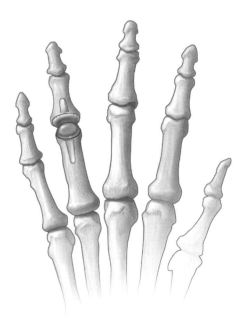

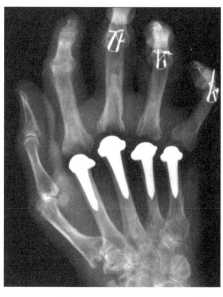

This illustration shows an artificial joint implant in the ring finger.

This X-ray shows the hand of a person with rheumatoid arthritis who has received four knuckle joint implants.

A hand for Laura

I used to make a living with my hands. I was a factory welder, making auto parts.

Nine-and-a-half years into the job, when I was 39, I woke up one spring morning with a foot aching horribly. I went to my family doctor, who diagnosed tendinitis and gave me steroids. But within a week, the pain had spread to joints throughout my body: both feet, hands, wrists, knees, everywhere. I went back to the doctor and said, "Tell me this isn't arthritis." For I was suffering from what I remember my grandmother had. My blood tested positive for rheumatoid arthritis.

I pushed myself at work and managed to hang on for six more months, long enough to qualify for a pension. But within three years after the pain had started, my hands had become nearly worthless. I remember going to the grocery store one day and not being able to open the door. It was too heavy. I turned around and cried all the way home.

Even drinking a glass of water became tough; I had to hold it with the heels of my hands. Eating out was too embarrassing. But with my family's help, I made adaptations around the house. My favorite was a foot pedal that opened the refrigerator. Another was a nail that my husband drove through a cutting board. I would stick a potato on the nail so that it wouldn't slip away when I cleaned or peeled it.

That's about the time I decided to replace the knuckle joints in all five fingers of my right hand. The doctor warned me that the new joints wouldn't work as well as the ones God gave me. But I sat there thinking that the ones God gave me didn't work at all.

It took a year before the fingers felt like they belonged to me. But now I have one hand that can do just about anything I need it to do. I can twist the key that starts the car — something I hadn't been able to do for years. I even hand painted a dozen sweat suits for Christmas presents.

Laura
Grand Rapids, Mich.

tears and prevent rupture of these tendons. Other surgical procedures help tighten or loosen tendons and ligaments in the hand
and wrist to decrease your pain and increase your mobility and
grip strength.

Synovectomy may help reduce pain in the wrists and fingers
caused by rheumatoid arthritis. Joint fusion can relieve pain and
improve stability in severely damaged finger and wrist joints. But
wrist fusion causes a decrease in hand mobility.

Hand and wrist joint replacements are performed less often than
hip and knee arthroplasties, partly because the joints are small, are
close to the skin and require precise repair of ligaments and tendons. The hand is also complex, with many moving parts. Because
more conservative procedures such as joint fusion and tendon
repairs produce favorable results, many surgeons reserve replacement for only the most severely damaged hand and wrist joints. In
the case of knuckle replacement surgery, some surgeons reserve the
procedure for people over age 50, who tend to use their hands less,
allowing the artificial knuckles to last longer.

If you have joint replacement surgery on your hand or wrist,
your hand will be placed in a splint for two to three weeks while
the soft tissues heal. You will then undergo an intense program of
physical therapy to retrain the tissues. Because there is so much
soft tissue reconstruction involved in wrist or finger arthroplasty,
physical therapy after surgery is essential.

Elbows

If medications and daily exercise aren't giving you enough relief
from arthritis pain in your elbow, you might consider other options.
Several surgical procedures can reduce your pain and increase the
range of motion in your elbow. Possibilities range from arthroscopic
procedures that require small incisions and short recovery times to
complete surgical replacement of your elbow joint.

Elbow surgery for arthritis is generally performed in one of two
ways. Open surgery refers to the traditional method of operating —
accessing the target site through a large incision in the arm. Open
surgery on the elbow is widely available, and surgeons have been
doing it for years.

The other option is arthroscopic surgery. In arthroscopic elbow surgery, your surgeon makes small incisions though which a tiny camera is inserted in your elbow. Images from the camera are projected onto a monitor in the operating room. Your surgeon can see into the joint area using the camera and performs the surgery using the images as a guide.

Arthroscopic elbow surgery offers the advantages of decreased risk of infection and less postoperative scarring. But it requires special expertise because the surgeon is moving the tiny camera and surgical tools within millimeters of nerves within your elbow. Also, if your elbow has deteriorated from arthritis, your risk of complications is increased. Depending on the stage of your arthritis, arthroscopic surgery might not be an option. Because arthroscopic elbow surgery is still evolving, the procedure isn't available at all medical centers.

The specific surgical procedure that's right for you will depend on several factors, including the type of arthritis — osteoarthritis or rheumatoid arthritis — and the condition of your elbow.

Synovectomy (sin-o-veck-TUH-mee), performed by itself or with bone resection, is usually the first choice in surgery for people with early stages of rheumatoid arthritis. It can help increase your elbow's range of motion and relieve pain. You and your doctor might consider synovectomy if you've tried medication and therapy for at least six months and you still have severe pain in your elbow.

The synovectomy procedure can be open or arthroscopic. Because arthroscopy uses high-powered optics and very small surgical instruments, and it allows your surgeon to see and access more of your joint, arthroscopic synovectomy is more thorough.

The synovium in your joints eventually grows back, which means that your elbow pain could return in a few years. But synovectomy can delay the need for more invasive surgical treatments, such as elbow replacement. Plus, medications can prevent your synovium from becoming inflamed again.

For osteoarthritis, debridement is usually the first surgery used after medications and physical therapy fail to bring relief from pain. Debridement also can be performed as an open surgery or arthroscopically.

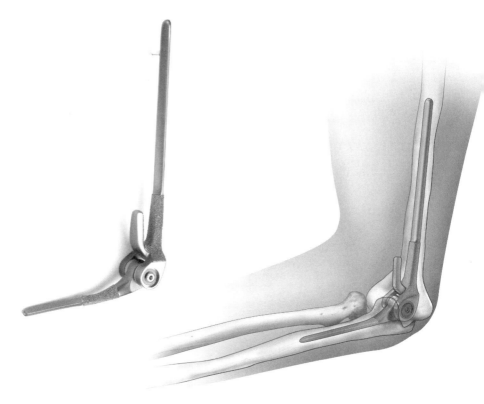

The hinged elbow implant shown here permits movement of the elbow in one plane (extending and flexing of the forearm). Another more complex elbow implant (not shown) also permits rotation of the forearm, similar to a normal joint.

Other surgical options for treating osteoarthritis or rheumatoid arthritis of the elbow include interposition arthroplasty, osteocapsular arthroplasty and elbow replacement, also called total elbow arthroplasty.

In interposition arthroplasty, which is an open surgery, your surgeon removes any bone spurs or loose pieces of bone. He or she then dislocates your elbow and stitches a piece of your skin or tendon — usually from your abdomen or Achilles tendon — in place between the bones that make up your elbow joint. This resurfaces the joint, keeping your bones from rubbing together, thereby reducing your pain.

The benefits of interposition arthroplasty may last up to 20 years. But you might need a total elbow replacement later in life.

If you're under age 60 and have severe arthritis, you might consider interposition arthroplasty. Generally, people younger than 60 aren't offered the option of elbow replacement surgery, so interposition arthroplasty is performed as an intermediate surgery between debridement or synovectomy and total joint replacement.

Osteocapsular arthroplasty, which is gradually replacing interposition arthroplasty, is a new arthroscopic procedure for arthritis of the elbow. A more thorough form of debridement, it includes the removal of bone spurs, loose bone and loose cartilage, as well as synovectomy and recontouring of bones that have become deformed or have deteriorated because of arthritis. Although osteocapsular arthroplasty can be extremely successful, it's also very difficult to perform. Because it's relatively new and requires substantial expertise, osteocapsular arthroplasty isn't widely available.

Total joint replacement of the elbow — also called total elbow arthroplasty — is usually reserved for people with advanced arthritis that hasn't responded to nonsurgical treatments and less aggressive surgical options. It's generally done in older adults — those 60 and older — and it isn't recommended for younger people unless other types of surgery have failed. If you have intolerable pain that doesn't respond to medication and your daily activities are limited by your arthritis, you might consider elbow replacement.

During elbow replacement surgery, your surgeon makes an incision in the back side of your elbow and moves muscles and nerves out of the way. He or she then removes parts of the bones in your elbow, reshapes the remaining bone to accept the artificial joint, and cements the metal prosthetic joint into place. Elbow implants are typically secured with a combination of cement and growth of bone into the implant (bone ingrowth). Replacing the diseased bones and tissue with the artificial joint, which is similar to a hinge, relieves pain and restores range of motion.

As with any surgery, elbow replacement carries the risk of infection and bleeding. Also, mechanical problems in the artificial joint, such as loosening of the implant or breakage, are more likely to occur in the elbow than in other joints because of the tremendous stress that the elbow undergoes. Injury to the nerves in your elbow is also possible.

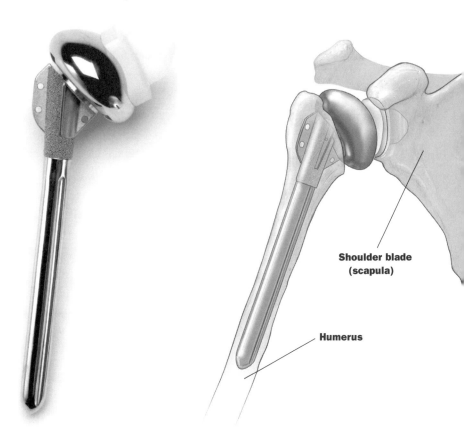

Shoulder blade
(scapula)

Humerus

The image at left shows an artificial shoulder joint as it would be positioned following surgery. At right is an illustration of a total shoulder replacement. The plastic component positioned against the ball of the artificial joint is anchored to the shoulder blade (scapula).

Elbow replacement can increase range of motion in your elbow and reduce pain. But your use of the new elbow is subject to severe limitations. After surgery, you shouldn't lift more than one or two pounds regularly, and lifting up to 10 pounds can only be done occasionally. Heavier lifting could damage the new joint or the bones holding it in place. These restrictions are in place for the life of your new joint.

Shoulders

Doctors usually recommend daily exercises or medications to treat arthritis of the shoulder. However, if pain and lack of motion persist after you've tried these options, it may be time to consider surgery. Joint replacement is the most common surgical procedure for arthritis of the shoulder. But there are also other surgical procedures to relieve shoulder pain that hasn't responded to more conservative measures.

If you have rheumatoid arthritis and the bones in your shoulder joint aren't damaged, a synovectomy might be all you need to restore motion and reduce pain. Synovectomy can be done with either an open or an arthroscopic surgery. Your synovium can grow back and become inflamed once again, but medications can usually prevent that from happening. Studies show that among people with rheumatoid arthritis of the shoulder who undergo synovectomy, up to 80 percent eventually have pain-free motion.

When bone or cartilage damage in your shoulder is more extensive, more aggressive surgery may be needed. Joint fusion, or arthrodesis, can reduce pain and offer long-term stability in joints that are more severely damaged. But because the fusion doesn't allow your joint to move, the procedure significantly reduces your ability to use your shoulder. Arthrodesis is less common today than it once was. You might be a candidate for this procedure if damage from arthritis makes it impossible for the muscles and tendons in your shoulder to support and hold an artificial shoulder joint in place or if you have had an infection of the shoulder joint with cartilage loss.

Osteocapsular arthroplasty is another surgical option for arthritis of the shoulder. During this procedure, your surgeon removes bone spurs and reshapes and smooths your shoulder joint's surfaces. This makes it easier for the bones in your shoulder to move without friction and pain. Your surgeon may perform this surgery arthroscopically by inserting a tiny camera (arthroscope) and special instruments into your joint though small incisions.

Total joint replacement (arthroplasty) is the most common type of shoulder surgery for arthritis. It can increase the range of motion in your shoulder, making it easier to move your arm. It also improves strength and reduces pain in your shoulder.

During total joint replacement, your surgeon removes the damaged parts of the bones that make up your shoulder joint and

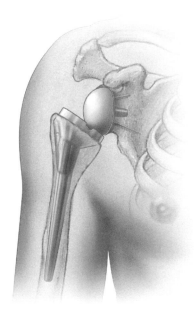

This illustration shows a reverse shoulder implant. The ball component is fixed to the shoulder blade (scapula), and the socket component is fixed to the upper arm (humerus).

replaces them with metal and plastic prostheses. Prostheses replace the ball-shaped top of your upper arm bone (humerus) and the cup-shaped glenoid cavity of your shoulder blade. Your surgeon might also clean up the area around your shoulder joint by removing any bone spurs (osteophytes) and the tissue that surrounds your joint (synovium), which can become inflamed and painful.

When performed by an experienced surgeon, total shoulder arthroplasty restores almost two-thirds of normal shoulder motion. In addition, studies show that between 70 percent to 90 percent of people who've had the procedure report no pain or only mild pain. But a longer rehabilitation period is necessary with shoulder replacement than with other types of joint replacements. Learning to use your new shoulder joint and recovering its strength may take several months. Fully regaining your strength and function may take up to a year. You have to diligently adhere to a prescribed set of exercises beginning the first day after surgery. Not sticking to the exercise regimen can lead to stiffness or instability and dissatisfaction with your new shoulder joint.

Although modern shoulder replacement surgery has been in common use for over 30 years, recent advances in technology and technique have made the procedure fairly safe and predictable. As with any surgery, though, you face a risk of infection and bleeding.

Most people are happy with their new shoulder joints, but complications can arise. A small number of total joint replacements — about 5 percent — eventually need to be replaced. The prostheses can loosen, requiring refitting. Sometimes, the shoulder becomes weak and unstable, which might require another joint replacement surgery.

If you're younger and want to use your shoulder more vigorously than possible with a complete joint replacement, you may want to consider a version of total joint replacement called hemiarthroplasty. In this procedure, only the ball-shaped top of your upper arm bone is replaced. The socket-shaped glenoid cavity of your shoulder blade may also be smoothed out, but a glenoid prosthesis isn't inserted. If you have a rotator cuff tear in addition to arthritis, you might also consider hemiarthroplasty.

Another option is reverse total shoulder arthroplasty. As its name implies, a reverse shoulder prosthesis is a turnabout from the typical artificial shoulder. Instead of the ball portion being attached to the upper arm bone and the cup portion being attached to the shoulder blade, the reverse prosthesis is placed so that the ball portion is attached to the socket of the shoulder blade. The cup portion is attached to the top of the upper arm bone.

The reverse shoulder prosthesis is most appropriate for people who have very difficult shoulder problems. These include having arthritis in the joint, along with extensive tears of multiple muscles and tendons that support the shoulder (rotator cuff), or having extensive rotator cuff tears and a failed previous shoulder joint replacement.

There's some concern about whether the reverse shoulder prosthesis, which is relatively new, will develop unexpected mechanical problems or loosen over time. But the early results have been promising.

Hips

The daily demands you place on your hips to bear weight, walk, climb stairs, bend and twist make them your hardest-working

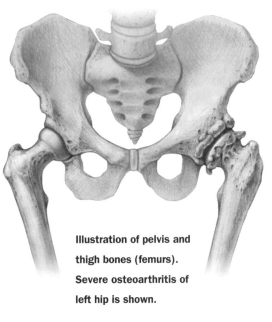

Illustration of pelvis and thigh bones (femurs). Severe osteoarthritis of left hip is shown.

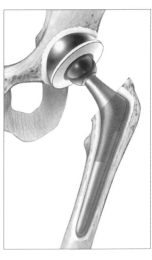

Left hip after total joint replacement. Components are cemented in place.

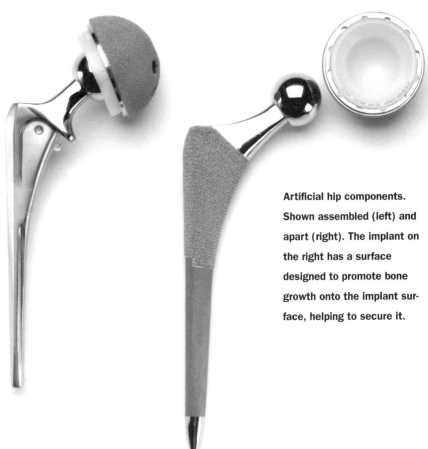

Artificial hip components. Shown assembled (left) and apart (right). The implant on the right has a surface designed to promote bone growth onto the implant surface, helping to secure it.

joints. When losing weight, taking medications, limiting your activity and using a cane fail to provide relief, a hip operation may be the answer.

Osteotomy — a surgery that cuts away bone — is occasionally used to help reduce hip pain. During this procedure, your surgeon gets rid of some of the diseased bone and tissue and returns the joint to its proper position. This helps evenly distribute your weight and, for some people, brings pain relief and improved function of the hip joint. But osteotomy isn't the answer for everyone. Recovery takes time, up to six to 12 months, and after surgery the hip may continue to deteriorate, causing a need for further treatment.

Joint fusion, or arthrodesis of the hip, is another surgical option. During this procedure, your surgeon creates a union between the round upper end of your thighbone (femur) and the socket in your pelvic bone (acetabulum), eliminating all motion. Those best suited to this procedure are young people whose activity level may place too much stress on an artificial joint, such as people who perform manual labor or participate in demanding sports.

Hip replacement surgery, also called total hip arthroplasty, is by far the most successful surgical procedure for treating advanced arthritis of the hip. It's also one of the most common joint replacement surgeries, with more than 190,000 done annually in the United States.

The surgery involves replacing the femoral head — the "ball" of your thighbone — with a metal ball. The metal ball attaches to a metal stem that fits into your thighbone. A plastic and metal socket is implanted into your pelvic bone to replace the damaged socket. The prosthetic parts, which mimic the natural design of your hip, fit together and function like a normal hip joint (see page 152).

Artificial hip joints come in many varieties. Generally your surgeon decides which hip joint is the best for you. Materials used in making the prostheses include a combination of durable, wear-resistant plastic and metals, including stainless steel and titanium. Implants are biocompatible — meaning they're designed to be accepted by your body — and they're made to resist corrosion, degradation and wear.

Some artificial hip joints are cemented, meaning that they're held in place by a bonding material called bone cement or methyl-methacrylate. Others are uncemented, meaning that they're held in place by new bone growing into part of the prosthesis over time. No hard and fast rules dictate whether cemented or uncemented fixation should be used. In general, uncemented fixation is used in people age 50 and younger who have good bone quality. Cemented fixation is used for people age 70 and older or younger people with compromised health or poor bone quality. For people between ages 50 and 70, it's not uncommon for hybrid fixation to be used, in which the socket is fixed without cement and the stem is fixed with cement.

Hip replacement surgery usually takes two to three hours, during which time you'll be under general or regional anesthesia. During the operation, your thighbone is separated from the socket. Working between the large hip muscles, the diseased or damaged bone and tissue is removed, leaving healthy bone and tissue intact. Next, the artificial socket is pressed into place. The top end of the thighbone is hollowed out to allow insertion of the metal stem with the attached ball. The ball and the socket join to form the new hip joint. Before closing the incision, your surgeon checks the alignment of the new joint.

A relatively new approach to managing pain following hip replacement and other joint replacement surgery is the use of a peripheral nerve catheter. The catheter is placed on the day of surgery and remains in place for 48 hours. It supplies medication directly to the nerves in the region of the joint to be replaced, effectively numbing the area. The technique reduces or eliminates uncomfortable side effects from narcotic pain medications normally used in such cases. It has also reduced recovery time following surgery. The technique is commonly used at Mayo Clinic and is currently available at only a few institutions around the United States.

You will stay in the hospital for a few days while you recover. As early as the day after your surgery, you may be encouraged to sit up and even try walking with crutches or a walker. A physical therapist may help you with some exercises that you can do in the hospital and at home to speed recovery. Before you leave the hospital, you and your caregivers will learn the best way for you to dress, sit down in a chair, get out of bed, use the toilet and climb stairs.

Hip replacement surgery is generally safe but, as with any surgery, complications can occur. Although some complications are serious, most can be treated successfully. In rare circumstances, complications can include blood clots, dislocation, infection, loosening, breakage of the prosthesis, change in leg length or joint stiffening.

Activity and exercise must be a regular part of your day to regain the use of your joint and muscles. Your physical therapist will recommend strengthening and mobility exercises and will help you learn how to use a walking aid, such as a walker or crutches. As therapy progresses, you'll gradually increase the weight you put on your leg until you're able to walk without assistance.

About six to eight weeks after surgery, you'll have a follow-up appointment with your surgeon to make sure your hip is healing properly. If recovery is progressing well, most people resume their normal activities by this time — even if in a limited fashion.

The odds of a successful recovery are in your favor — hip replacement surgery is successful more than 90 percent of the time. You can expect to be pain-free for 10 to 15 years after surgery. But don't expect to do things that you couldn't do before surgery. High-impact activities — such as running or playing basketball — may never get your doctor's approval. But in time, you may be able to swim, play golf, walk or ride a bike comfortably.

Hip replacement used to be an option primarily for adults age 60 and older. But improved technology has made strong and longer-lasting artificial joints that are feasible for more active people, including younger people. However, active people face the possibility of another surgery to replace worn out artificial hip joints after 15 or 20 years. A repeated hip replacement surgery, also called revision surgery, is more difficult and often isn't as successful as the original surgery.

One noteworthy change in hip replacement surgery is the recent development of less invasive and minimally invasive surgical tech-

niques. Some surgeons are doing "mini-hips" through one relatively small incision — about 3 ½ inches. Others use two-incision techniques with even shorter incisions. Accessing the hip joint through
two smaller incisions allows surgeons to minimize the cutting of
muscles, ligaments and tendons.

These newer, less invasive procedures aren't right for everyone.
The procedures are much more technically demanding than traditional hip replacement, and there can be complications, such as dislocated hips, bone fractures and nerve and blood vessel injuries.
And because these procedures are relatively new, there are no studies demonstrating long-term outcomes. Some short-term studies
have shown that people who undergo minimally invasive hip
replacement have an easier and less painful recovery, spend less
time in the hospital and have fewer complications. But other studies haven't found this. More studies and longer follow-up are needed to evaluate minimally invasive techniques.

Knees

Several surgical options are available to relieve knee pain and
restore mobility. Arthroscopic debridement is frequently used to
repair cartilage tears or remove loose tissue fragments. This may be
a good approach if you're young or middle-aged and have arthritis
as the result of sports injuries.

Synovectomy can decrease pain and swelling in people with
rheumatoid arthritis whose cartilage is not significantly damaged.
Although it doesn't appear to slow the progression of the disease,
synovectomy may delay the need for a total joint replacement in
younger people. Because the knee joint is relatively large, surgeons
typically use an arthroscope to perform this procedure. Using this
device, the surgeon can view the joint and remove the diseased tissue with other instruments. Arthroscopic synovectomy requires a
much smaller incision than a traditional operation, so recovery is
usually much quicker.

Doctors sometimes recommend osteotomy — the surgical
removal of bone — to slow cartilage damage in the knees and
relieve pain. By trimming and repositioning the leg bones, weight
can be more evenly distributed across your knee joint and correct

curvature or bowing in the lower leg bones caused by osteoarthritis. Surgeons typically recommend this procedure for younger, more active people.

Joint fusion, or arthrodesis of the knee, is an option for people who aren't candidates for knee replacement surgery, perhaps because of their age, activity level or weight, or if an artificial knee becomes infected and can't be salvaged. Even though fusion limits knee motion, it allows you to bear weight on your leg without pain.

Knee replacement surgery — also known as total knee arthroplasty — can help relieve pain and restore function in severely diseased knee joints. In the 1950s, the first artificial knees were little more than crude hinges. Now that more than 350,000 knee replacement surgeries are performed each year, you and your doctor can choose from a wide variety of designs that take into account your age, weight, activity level and overall health. Most attempt to replicate your knee's natural ability to roll and glide as it bends.

Although most people who undergo knee replacement are age 55 or older, surgeons occasionally replace knees in people who are younger. The active lifestyles of younger people may cause greater wear and stress on the artificial knee, requiring it to be replaced in the future.

During knee replacement surgery, your surgeon cuts away damaged bone and cartilage from your thighbone, shinbone and kneecap and replaces it with an artificial joint (prostheses) made of metal alloys, high-grade plastics and polymers.

One of the largest parts of an artificial knee joint is made of metal alloy and attaches to the end of the thighbone (femur) where diseased bone has been removed. Another major component, also of metal alloy, resembles a tray on a pedestal. The pedestal portion of this component is anchored into the shaft of your shinbone (tibia). The platform of the tray has a surface of high-density plastic. It provides a resting place for the metal component attached to your femur. The plastic acts as the joint's new cartilage. Some artificial knee joints also include another small component — a circular piece of plastic that attaches to your kneecap to replace cartilage or diseased bone.

Front view   **Side view**

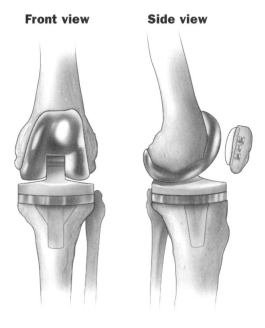

Total knee arthroplasty with components in place. A plastic component is fixed to the backside of the kneecap (patella).

Artificial knee implant

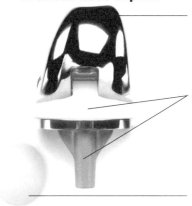

Metal femoral component. Attaches to the thighbone (femur).

Plastic and metal tibial components. Attach to the shinbone (tibia).

Kneecap (patellar) component

Some artificial knee joints are cemented, meaning that they're held in place by a bonding material called bone cement (methylmethacrylate). Others are uncemented, meaning that they're held in place by new bone growing into part of the prosthesis over time. Mayo Clinic surgeons believe that cemented prostheses have less chance of early loosening and developing other problems.

Knee replacement surgery usually takes about two hours, during which time you'll be under general or regional anesthesia.

During the procedure, your knee is in a bent position so that all surfaces of the joint are fully exposed. After making an incision between 6 and 12 inches in length, the muscles, kneecap and connective tissues are moved aside, and the damaged bone and cartilage is cut away. The existing connective tissues are also realigned to hold the joint together after the prosthesis is in place. Leg bones damaged by arthritis also may need to be realigned.

Your surgeon takes measurements to ensure a good fit for your new prosthesis and smooths your bones' rough edges. The prosthesis is then inserted. Before closing the incision, your surgeon bends and rotates your knee, testing and balancing it to ensure that it functions properly.

You will likely stay in the hospital for several days. You may feel some pain, but medications can help control it. The day after surgery, a physical therapist may help you to exercise your new knee. To help regain movement, you may use a device called a continuous passive motion machine, which slowly moves your knee while you're in bed. As with any surgery, knee replacement surgery carries risk of potentially life-threatening infection, heart attack and stroke. Other risks include knee-joint infection, nerve damage and the possibility that your new knee could break or become dislocated.

Blood clots in the leg vein (thrombophlebitis) are a major concern with knee replacement surgery, so blood thinners are commonly used to help prevent them. During the hospital stay, you'll be encouraged to move your foot and ankle, which increases blood flow to your leg muscles and helps prevent swelling and blood clots. You may need to receive blood thinners and wear support hose or compression boots to further protect against swelling and clotting.

During the first few weeks after surgery, your physical activity program typically includes a graduated walking program — first indoors, then outdoors — and the knee-strengthening exercises you learned from the hospital physical therapist. You may also be advised to slowly resume other normal household activities, including walking up and down stairs. Three to six weeks after the procedure — depending on your doctor's assessment — you generally can resume most normal daily activities such as shopping and

Getting a new hip or knee? Plan ahead for your recovery

Expect your recovery from knee or hip replacement surgery to take some time. It may be several months before you can resume all of your normal activities.

To make things easier on yourself, plan for your return home before you go in for surgery. Try these tips:

- Ask someone — a family member, friend or neighbor — to help you get home from the hospital and to assist you for a week or two after you're discharged. Or you might arrange for a temporary caretaker or for a stay at a step-down care facility during this time.
- Install safety bars or a secure handrail in your shower or bath and arrange for a toilet-seat riser with arms if you have a low toilet. Try a stable bench or chair for your shower.
- Make sure the handrails along your stairways are secure.
- If possible, arrange your bedroom with extra space around the bed to allow room to get in and out while using crutches, a walker or a cane. If your bedroom is up or down a flight of stairs, temporarily move your bed to a room on the main level of your home.
- Rearrange your kitchen so that you can easily reach utensils. Place them in convenient locations to minimize bending or stretching.
- Prepare some meals in advance and freeze them.
- Ask your mail and newspaper carriers to deliver to your door, if possible.
- Request a visit from your clergy person or spiritual adviser while you recover, if you wish.
- Leave your home clean and orderly so that you won't need to clean it when you return.
- Remove all throw rugs, cords and clutter from traffic paths.
- Consider placing a clean plastic trash bag on the car seat to make it easier to turn your body once you're seated.
- Be sure to get instructions on how best to lie down and sit up in bed.

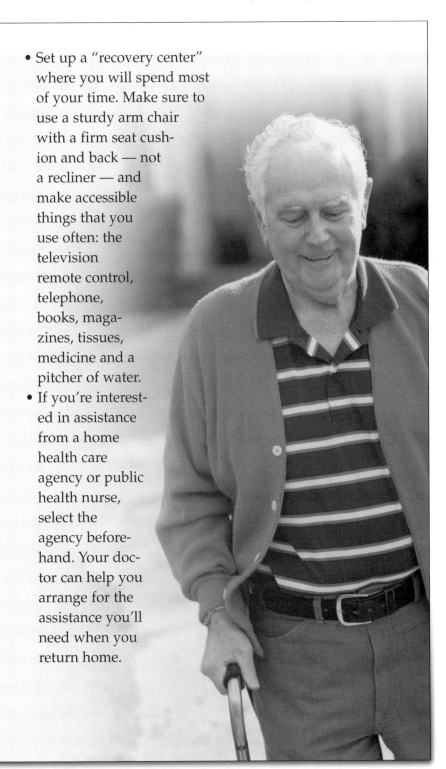

- Set up a "recovery center" where you will spend most of your time. Make sure to use a sturdy arm chair with a firm seat cushion and back — not a recliner — and make accessible things that you use often: the television remote control, telephone, books, magazines, tissues, medicine and a pitcher of water.
- If you're interested in assistance from a home health care agency or public health nurse, select the agency beforehand. Your doctor can help you arrange for the assistance you'll need when you return home.

light housekeeping. Driving is generally possible in four to six weeks if you can bend your knee far enough to sit in a car and you have enough muscle control to properly operate the brakes and accelerator.

About 90 percent of people who have a total knee replacement experience significant pain relief, improved mobility and a better overall quality of life. High-impact activities increase the risk of knee failure. To reduce your risk, avoid activities such as jogging or running, contact or jumping sports, high-impact aerobics, vigorous walking or hiking, skiing, tennis, repetitive lifting of objects exceeding 50 pounds, and repetitive aerobic stair climbing. After you've recovered, you can enjoy a variety of low-impact activities, such as recreational walking, swimming, golf, recreational biking and ballroom dancing.

If only a part of your knee is involved with arthritis, your doctor may suggest an implant to replace just the damaged part of your knee. This procedure, called partial knee replacement, is less extensive and will usually allow for faster recovery. The knee also will feel more like your natural knee. To determine whether you are a candidate for this procedure, your surgeon will need to be sure that other parts of your knee joint aren't affected by arthritis. Usually this can be determined by X-rays and other images. In some cases, your doctor may not be able to make this decision until the time of surgery.

Since the late 1990s, some surgeons have offered a minimally invasive total knee replacement procedure. This procedure involves making a smaller incision of four to five inches instead of the typical 10 to 12 inches. This reduces the trauma to muscles and tendons, resulting in a shorter hospital stay, a faster recovery and less scarring. More research into the long-term effects of this method is necessary to know whether this newer procedure is as safe and effective as standard total knee replacement. Researchers may not have an answer for another 10 to 15 years.

Ankles and feet

Like your hips and knees, your ankles and feet are weight-bearing joints that help carry you through your day. Various operations are

Your body's joints

Your body has several types of joints:

- **Fixed.** These joints don't move. They absorb shock to help prevent bones from breaking. Fixed joints in your skull protect sensitive brain tissue underneath.
- **Hinge.** Like the hinge in a doorway, your knee joints let you move forward and backward.
- **Pivot.** These joints allow a rotating movement. Your elbow has both hinge and pivot joints.
- **Ball-and-socket.** The large round end of a long bone fits into a hollow part of another bone. This makes swinging and rotating movements possible. You get the most movement from ball-and-socket joints in your hips and shoulders.

used to relieve pain and restore stability to these joints. Bone resection and repair of bunions or other bony growths in the feet can make walking and standing less painful.

Removal of cartilage and bony protrusions (debridement) and the surgical removal of bone (osteotomy) to realign the ankle can provide temporary relief from pain and can delay the need for more extensive surgery, perhaps for several years. These procedures can be done either as open surgery or arthroscopically, but the arthroscopic procedure is more common. For people who have rheumatoid arthritis of the forefoot, removal of synovial membrane tissue (synovectomy) early on may provide relief before cartilage becomes badly eroded. Research shows that for best results, synovectomy should be combined with immunosuppressive drug therapy.

If your symptoms are severe, your surgeon may recommend fusing the bones in your feet or ankle (arthrodesis) to improve stability and reduce pain. Although arthrodesis of the ankle eventually causes arthritic changes in the other joints of the foot, it remains the standard treatment for arthritis of the ankle, particularly if the condition has caused a severe deformity. The procedure also may be a good option if you're younger or middle-aged and want to resume high-impact sports or other strenuous activities.

Ankle and foot joint replacements are still rather new procedures that aren't widely used, partly because they lack a strong
record of success. Newer implant designs have reduced some of
the problems seen previously, such as wound complications and
persistent postoperative pain. But they haven't eliminated them
entirely. The life span of a current artificial ankle appears to be
about 10 years. Salvage after the joint fails remains a challenging
problem.

Preparing for your surgery

You and your surgeon will decide when you need to be admitted to
the hospital before your operation. Planning for meals, housekeeping and other assistance can help you cope with the change in
activity level you may experience after your operation.

Be sure to review your medications with your surgeon or family physician several weeks before your operation. Many surgeons
ask their patients to discontinue the use of aspirin and other nonsteroidal anti-inflammatory drugs (NSAIDs) up to a week before
the operation to minimize the risk of bleeding. Acetaminophen
(Tylenol, others) can usually be substituted for pain control if necessary. If you're taking methotrexate or other similar drugs, such
as azathioprine (Imuran) or cyclosporine (Sandimmune, Neoral),
for rheumatoid arthritis or the new biologic agents (Enbrel,
Humera, Remicade), your physician or surgeon probably will ask
you to stop taking it one or more weeks before the operation to
minimize the risk of infection. You can start again one or two
weeks afterward.

Potential risks and complications
You'll be monitored closely during and after the procedure to
reduce the chance of problems such as infection, blood loss, heart
attack or a blood clot in the lung. Other rare but possible complications are nerve and blood vessel injury, joint dislocation, bone loss
(with arthroplasty), and even death. Here's more on some of the
more common risks:

- Joint operation often requires a blood transfusion. The vast majority of people who receive transfusions have no adverse reactions. Still, the safest blood is your own. Your immune system will not react to your blood, and you cannot give yourself an infection.

  Use of a person's own blood, also known as autologous transfusion, has become common. When planning an elective operation, you can have units of your own blood drawn ahead of time. Usually, you give it about once a week over a period of a few weeks in advance of your operation. Your blood is stored and used as necessary to replace blood lost during the operation. National trends indicate that fewer surgical patients in the United States are donating their own blood before surgery. Nevertheless, the practice is recommended if you'll be undergoing a surgical procedure with substantial anticipated blood loss, such as total joint replacement surgery.

- Over the long term, the site of artificial joint implants is susceptible to infection. Bacteria can travel through your bloodstream and infect the surgical site, even years after the surgery. Notify your doctor immediately if you notice such warning signs as a fever greater than 100 F, shaking chills, drainage from the surgical site, and increasing redness, tenderness, swelling and pain around the artificial joint. If antibiotics fail to clear up the infection, you usually need one surgery to remove the infected joint and another surgery to install a new one. To reduce the risk of implant infection, your doctor may prescribe a course of antibiotics each time you have dental work, a gynecological exam, oral or certain other types of surgery, a catheterization, or a bacterial infection.

- Implants may also loosen or wear out with time, but improved designs and surgical techniques have prolonged the life of replacement joints. Rarely, an implanted artificial hip joint dislocates with certain movements or, more often, an injury. If you have rheumatoid arthritis in other joints, excessive stress on them in the postoperative period while you're protecting the operated joint may cause a flare-up.

Your hospital stay

The length of your hospital stay will depend on many factors, including the type of joint operation you have, your age and overall health and whether you experience any surgical complications.

After the procedure, your surgical care team will monitor your vital signs, alertness, and pain or comfort level and adjust your medications accordingly. Your doctor may prescribe antibiotics to prevent infection and anticoagulant medication to prevent blood clots.

Procedures that use only small incisions and local anesthesia, such as arthroscopic debridement and arthroscopic synovectomy, frequently do not require an overnight stay in the hospital.

In the 1960s, people stayed in bed for two to three weeks after a hip operation. Today, physical therapy begins almost immediately after most joint procedures, and hospital stays are shorter. Even though you may require assistance at first, you can probably expect to be up and out of your hospital bed several times daily. Remarkably, most people leave the hospital about three to six days after total joint replacement.

Rehabilitation

Exercise and rest are both important elements in recovery, so it's essential to follow the activity guidelines established by your surgeon or physical therapist. If you don't do your exercises, you can end up with a stiff, painful joint.

Physical therapists can help you learn the proper way to use and protect your new or altered joint. Exercise can improve joint motion, strengthen the muscles around your joint, reduce pain and help you improve your mobility. You may need to learn how to use assistive devices such as a walker, a cane or crutches to guard against falls or other injuries while your muscles and surgical site heal.

Occupational therapists can help you become independent in activities of daily living and instruct you in the use of assistive devices such as dressing aids, grab bars, a raised toilet seat and a bath bench. The goal of rehabilitation is for you to become as independent in your care and activities as possible.

Depending on your age, physical condition and home situation, your surgeon may recommend a short stay in a rehabilitation center to allow you to focus on your recovery before returning home.

Recovery at home

Continuing your recommended exercises at home will help you recover more quickly. Your doctor and physical therapist can tell you when you'll be able to return to your favorite activities and identify positions or activities to avoid. If your operation involved weight-bearing joints, you'll probably need to use crutches or a walker and then a cane for a while after you return to your home. If you have difficulty getting along at home, your doctor may recommend in-home visits by a physical or occupational therapist.

Joint infection may still be a risk after leaving the hospital. Make sure you contact your physician if you have a fever, if your incision opens or if you notice any increase in pain, tenderness, swelling, redness, warmth or drainage near the surgical site. Also watch for signs of circulation problems near your joint, such as numbness or tingling, or changes in color or temperature in your limbs.

Life after recovery

Full recovery from a joint operation may take only a few weeks for some tendon, ligament or cartilage repairs. Some types of joint fusion, osteotomy or joint replacements can require a few months to a full year of recovery before your bones heal fully and you regain your strength, stability and mobility. But many people experience a reduction in pain and swelling, as well as easier movement, just days after the procedure. Your age, overall health and commitment to your rehabilitation program can play a role in how quickly you recover. Follow-up visits with your doctor also are important.

Although recovering from joint replacement may take time, implants give many people a new lease on life. Between 10 and 15 years after surgery, more than 90 percent of those with knee replacements continue to have good to excellent results. After more than three decades, cemented hip implants also have a track record: About 80 percent of people can still walk comfortably 20 years after surgery.

Even with a successful joint operation, you may need to avoid high-impact activities such as running, downhill skiing or tennis. But, depending on which joint was affected, you should be able to resume an active, full life.

Chapter 7

Complementary and alternative treatments

Conventional medicine has much to offer in helping you manage your arthritis. But standard arthritis medicines can't "cure" arthritis and may not completely control symptoms. Some treatments carry the risk of unwanted and potentially serious side effects, especially after long-term use. In light of these issues, many people with arthritis understandably turn to other methods or treatments to help relieve pain and other symptoms.

Complementary and alternative medicine (CAM) encompasses a broad and diverse range of systems, practices and products that aren't typically part of conventional or mainstream medical practice. Complementary medicine is defined as treatments used along with conventional medical treatments. An example would be using an herbal product or self-hypnosis along with a standard pain medication to relieve pain. Alternative medicine is defined as treatments used in place of conventional medicine. An example might be seeing a homeopath instead of a medical doctor.

If you've tried some form of complementary or alternative medicine, you're not alone. A National Institutes of Health (NIH) 2002 survey of 31,000 adults in the United States found that 36 percent had used some form of CAM in the past year. Not surprisingly, the most common problems for which people sought CAM treatments involved conditions that conventional medicine hasn't been able to cure, such as back pain, head colds and anxiety. Pain is a powerful motivator to find some form of treatment that provides relief. In one survey of people with rheumatic disease, more than 60 percent had used some type of alternative care.

The list of what's considered complementary or alternative changes as new approaches to health care emerge and CAM therapies that are proved safe and effective become part of mainstream health care. Indeed, many hospitals, doctors and health insurers are integrating a variety of CAM treatments into their services. A trend toward integrative medicine, which combines conventional and CAM therapies, is increasing.

Acceptance of a treatment within the mainstream medical community is based in large part on scientific evidence. Some CAM therapies are backed by reliable scientific research. But the effectiveness and safety of the majority of CAM methods haven't been studied extensively using scientific methods. The stated effects of many CAM therapies are based on anecdotal evidence and theory rather than controlled studies. For these reasons, some doctors just don't know enough about CAM to endorse it. Nonetheless, a growing body of evidence indicates that some CAM practices have a role in treating some diseases. Several CAM techniques are recognized as helpful in managing chronic pain in some people.

For people with arthritis and other diseases that cause chronic pain, alternative treatments can provide a sense of control and self-direction. The desire to feel better and stay active is a strong incentive to seek treatments beyond conventional medicine. But it's also important to be aware of misleading claims and possible risks of some CAM therapies. This chapter provides an overview of many CAM treatments that are used for arthritis. It may help you sort out what's hype and what's helpful.

Types of complementary and alternative medicine

Some complementary and alternative medicine approaches share basic principles with Western medicine, but others don't. Many of these therapies have been practiced for thousands of years.

The National Center for Complementary and Alternative Medicine, a division of the National Institutes of Health, groups CAM treatments into five broad categories:

- Alternative medical and healing systems. These are complete systems of theory and practice that stem from a particular philosophy or lifestyle. Many of these systems, such as acupuncture and ayurveda, developed before conventional Western medicine.
- Biologically based practices. These use ingredients or substances found in nature, such as herbs, foods or vitamins (in doses different from those used in conventional medicine).
- Energy therapies. These techniques and practices involve the use of energy fields. They may be based on the belief that energy fields (biofields) surround and penetrate your body, or on the unconventional use of electromagnetic fields.
- Manipulative and body-based practices. These techniques, such as massage or chiropractic, involve physically manipulating, moving or adjusting parts of the body.
- Mind-body interventions. These methods, such as meditation and guided imagery, promote healing by enhancing the mind's ability to influence the body.

Each category includes several types of CAM. Many of these are used — with varying degrees of success — to treat arthritis.

Alternative medical and healing systems

Alternative medical systems often emphasize the whole person — mind, body and spirit — in treating and preventing disease. Traditional Asian, American Indian and Pacific Islander medicine and practices fall into this category.

In the United States, alternative medical systems haven't been used often to treat arthritis. But some evidence suggests a possible benefit from acupuncture, ayurvedic herbs and homeopathy.

Acupuncture

Originating in China more than 2,500 years ago, acupuncture is one of the oldest forms of medicine in the world. This system of care is based on the theory that stimulating specific points in the body allows the free flow of qi, or chi (pronounced chee), the Chinese word for energy or life force. Traditional acupuncturists believe that pain is reduced and health is restored when qi flows without obstruction along pathways called meridians that run throughout your body.

These meridians are accessible through approximately 400 different acupuncture points. By inserting extremely thin needles into acupuncture points in various combinations, acupuncture practitioners aim to rebalance your energy flow. Although the most common way of stimulating acupuncture points is with needles, other techniques can be used. For example, in acupressure, practitioners use their fingers instead of needles to apply pressure to acupuncture points.

During a typical acupuncture session, the practitioner inserts anywhere from one to 40 disposable, sterilized stainless steel needles for 15 to 40 minutes. He or she may also manipulate the needles manually or by electrical stimulation or heat.

Research indicates that acupuncture stimulates your body's own morphine-like painkilling chemicals, called endorphins. Acupuncture may be particularly appealing to people who can't tolerate side effects associated with long-term use of nonsteroidal anti-inflammatory drugs (NSAIDs).

A growing body of evidence supports the use of acupuncture in certain situations. For example, the National Institutes of Health found that acupuncture provides pain relief and improves function for people with osteoarthritis of the knee, based on the results of a large, well-designed study involving 570 people. Participants, who were age 50 and older and had osteoarthritis of the knee, were randomly assigned to receive one of three treatments: acupuncture, sham acupuncture or a self-help program. People receiving acupuncture had a significant decrease in pain and improvement in function compared with the sham and control groups. The researchers suggest that acupuncture can serve as an effective complement to standard care for people with knee osteoarthritis. Other clinical trials of acupuncture for osteoarthritis are under way.

Acupuncture may also help people with other pain-related conditions, such as low back pain or fibromyalgia. Future research may better define whether people with other types of arthritis are likely to benefit from acupuncture.

Some medical doctors remain skeptical about the effectiveness of acupuncture, because studies have shown that some people experience pain relief regardless of where the needles are placed. In addition, acupuncture meridians don't appear to correspond to physical structures or systems in the body, such as nerve or blood circulation pathways. The acceptance of a treatment that's based on theories that aren't familiar in Western medicine can be difficult.

Nonetheless, public use and awareness of acupuncture has grown, and it's becoming more available in conventional medical settings.

Acupuncture is generally a low-risk treatment. Most people feel little or no pain as the needles are inserted. Once the needles are in place, you shouldn't feel any pain.

Ayurvedic medicine

Ayurveda is an alternative medicine system that dates back 5,000 years to ancient India. The aim of ayurvedic medicine is to promote health rather than fight disease, by emphasizing harmony in body, mind and spirit. Treatment is individualized and may include nutrition, fasting, exercise, herbs, meditation and massage.

Few scientific studies have examined the use of ayurveda in treating arthritis. The little research that has been done has focused mostly on the herbal medicine aspect of ayurveda and not the other parts of it. Some studies have shown a possible benefit of various ayurvedic herbal mixtures for osteoarthritis and rheumatoid arthritis. Ayurvedic herbs may help reduce pain and stiffness, but more and better-designed research is needed to confirm the preliminary findings.

Homeopathic medicine

Homeopathy was developed by German physician Samuel Hahnemann in the late 18th century and is practiced around the globe. According to Hahnemann's law of similars, or "like cures like," if a substance causes you to develop certain symptoms when you're healthy, a small dose of this substance can treat illnesses that cause similar symptoms. Most homeopathic treatments are highly diluted preparations of natural substances, such as plants and minerals.

Scientific research hasn't yet explained how homeopathic medicines might work. Because most homeopathic medicines are so diluted that they contain virtually no molecules of the active substances, some scientists are skeptical about their effectiveness. A small number of studies have looked at the use of homeopathy for arthritis. While some trials showed that homeopathic treatments were twice as effective as a placebo (inactive treatment) in reducing pain and inflammation, most studies were of poor quality, making firm conclusions difficult.

Although traditional medical training isn't required, some homeopaths are physicians or other types of licensed health care providers, such as chiropractors, nurses or pharmacists. Regulation and licensure varies from state to state.

Biologically based treatments

Among the various forms of CAM, biologically based therapies make up the largest category. They encompass a wide range of ingredients found in nature, including herbs, vitamins, minerals, amino acids, animal extracts and enzymes. Other than prayer, natural products are the most commonly used form of CAM. Almost 20 percent of U.S. adults use natural products.

Herbal treatments have been used for thousands of years. Many of today's conventional medicines — including digoxin, used to treat congestive heart failure, and quinine, used to treat malaria — began as folk medicines. And scientists continue to discover new medicines derived from plants.

Outside conventional medicine, herbal preparations are sold as alternative pain relievers and inflammation fighters for both rheumatoid arthritis and osteoarthritis. Given the past success of medications derived from plants, research may someday help carve a niche for herbal treatments in the fight against arthritis symptoms.

The U.S. government defines a dietary supplement as a product (other than tobacco) taken by mouth that contains a "dietary ingredient" intended to supplement the diet. In addition to herbs, dietary ingredients include vitamins, minerals, amino acids, enzymes and other substances.

Many people trust in herbal medicine and dietary products because they are "natural." Remember, though, that natural doesn't necessarily mean that these products are safe or free of side effects. (See page 194 for tips on how to evaluate these remedies.) In addition, even the term "natural" doesn't have a universally accepted definition. Many supplements contain powerful substances that can be toxic or interfere with other medications. Because these products are subject to very limited regulatory oversight, it's difficult to tell which ones have been proved effective and how to use them safely. Different brands of the same herb may contain varying amounts of the "active" ingredient. For these reasons, talk to your doctor before you take any herbal preparation or dietary supplement.

Aromatherapy

This ancient form of healing uses essential oils (extracts or essences) from flowers, herbs and trees to promote health and beauty. Practitioners believe these oils can help treat various illnesses, including arthritis pain and inflammation, when massaged into your skin or inhaled. Used more widely in Europe than in the United States, aromatherapy treatments and products are found in stores that sell natural health products.

While many modern medications have come from plant extracts, more study is needed to determine whether any medicinal benefits are associated with the plant oils used in aromatherapy. No solid scientific research has been done on the use of aromatherapy for arthritis.

Avocado-soybean unsaponifiables

Avocado-soybean unsaponifiables (ASU) is a dietary supplement derived from avocado and soybean oils. Available evidence suggests that ASU is an effective treatment for osteoarthritis. In three clinical trials involving 587 people with osteoarthritis of the hip or knee, taking 300 milligrams of ASU daily provided relief from symptoms and reduced the need for nonsteroidal anti-inflammatory drugs.

In addition to reducing knee and hip pain and inflammation, ASU is thought by some to possibly slow structural damage to the hip joint.

ASU appears to be safe, with few side effects, though mild gastrointestinal discomfort is possible. This supplement may be a good option to try for people who are concerned about side effects of NSAIDs or can't tolerate them.

Bee venom

The belief that honeybee venom has curative powers has been around for centuries. Some people theorize that enzymes in bee venom can relieve symptoms of rheumatoid arthritis by fighting inflammation. Another hypothesis is that bee venom causes your body to increase its production of steroids, which may help relieve symptoms.

In bee venom therapy, purified bee venom is injected under your skin near problem joints. Bee venom acupuncture is a form of acupuncture in which diluted bee venom is administered with needles into acupuncture points.

A few early studies seemed to find a benefit of injected bee venom or bee venom acupuncture in treating arthritis. In the little scientific research that's been conducted, however, results have been conflicting. Large studies involving people (clinical trials) may help shed light on whether bee venom or one of its components can play a role in treating arthritis.

Bovine cartilage

Cartilage derived from cow tissues is thought to have anti-inflammatory effects, and some researchers think it can spur growth of new cartilage in people with osteoarthritis.

Injections of bovine cartilage given under the skin seem to help ease symptoms of both osteoarthritis and rheumatoid arthritis. A local allergic reaction (redness, swelling and itching) is possible, but other side effects are rare. More studies are needed to confirm the possible benefits and risks of this product.

Borage

The seeds of the borage plant are a rich source of gamma-linolenic acid (GLA), a fatty acid that's known to be moderately effective in reducing pain, joint tenderness and morning stiffness in people with rheumatoid arthritis. (GLA is discussed in more detail on page 179.) Borage seed oil may have some similar properties as NSAIDs. Oils made from black currant seeds and the evening primrose plant also contain GLA and are sometimes used for arthritis.

Some research suggests that taking borage seed oil in combination with conventional pain relievers or NSAIDs might decrease rheumatoid arthritis symptoms. But evidence to date doesn't show a clear benefit of taking black currant seed or evening primrose oil for arthritis symptoms.

Borage seed oil may cause soft stools, diarrhea, belching and bloating. If you use this product, make sure it is certified and labeled as hepatotoxic-pyrrolizidine alkaloid (PA)-free. Hepatotoxic PAs can cause severe liver disease and may possibly cause cancer.

Bromelain

Preliminary studies show that supplements of bromelain, a digestive enzyme extracted from pineapple, can reduce pain and inflammation. When combined with rutin (a citrus chemical) and trypsin (a pancreatic enzyme), bromelain may reduce the pain and swelling of arthritis as effectively as an NSAID. But better-quality studies are needed to confirm these findings. There isn't enough evidence to recommend use of bromelain for arthritis at this time.

Cat's claw

This dietary supplement is made from the root and bark of an Amazonian plant, *Uncaria tomentosa*, also known as cat's claw or the "life-giving vine of Peru." The supplement inhibits two inflammation-triggering substances — a type of prostaglandin and tumor necrosis factor-alpha (TNF-alpha). For osteoarthritis, cat's claw may relieve knee pain during physical activity but not during rest. For rheumatoid arthritis, cat's claw may have a modest effect in reducing the number of painful and swollen joints.

Further research is needed to establish the benefits and risks of cat's claw. Side effects may include headache, dizziness and vomiting. Cat's claw may lower your blood pressure, so if you take other blood pressure lowering (antihypertensive) drugs, talk to your doctor before taking this supplement.

Devil's claw

Devil's claw is widely marketed as an herbal remedy for osteoarthritis. The plant's scientific name is *Harpagophytum procumbens,* and it's claimed to have anti-inflammatory, analgesic and antioxidant properties. Several studies have shown that devil's claw reduces pain from osteoarthritis, especially hip and knee pain. A specific devil's claw extract, taken in a dose of 2.6 grams a day, seemed to improve pain relief when used with NSAIDs. Devil's claw has no known benefit for rheumatoid arthritis.

Side effects may include diarrhea and an increased risk of bleeding and bruising. Devil's claw may exacerbate the risk of gastrointestinal bleeding from NSAIDs or corticosteroids.

Dimethylsulfoxide

Dimethylsulfoxide (DMSO) is an industrial solvent, similar to turpentine, that is sold as a topical treatment for arthritis. Some evidence suggests that DMSO can relieve pain and reduce swelling when rubbed directly on the skin, but it may be no more effective than other topical, over-the-counter pain relief products.

Nearly 40 years of medical research on DMSO has yielded conflicting results. DMSO isn't approved by the Food and Drug Administration (FDA) for human use, except for treating a rare type of bladder inflammation.

Industrial-strength DMSO (sold in hardware stores) may contain poisonous contaminants that can penetrate the skin. Used topically, DMSO can cause sedation, headache, dizziness, drowsiness, nausea, vomiting, diarrhea, constipation, skins problems, dry or sore throat, cough, worsening of asthma, and a flu-like syndrome. For these reasons, arthritis experts don't recommend using this solvent as a treatment for arthritis.

Fish oil

Cold-water fish such as salmon, mackerel, herring, sardine and trout are high in polyunsaturated fats called omega-3 fatty acids. These fatty acids play an important role in many body functions and can help reduce inflammation.

Oil derived from these fish has been shown to improve pain, tender joints, morning stiffness and other symptoms in people with rheumatoid arthritis. Using fish oils might also allow people to reduce their use of NSAIDs. Studies haven't found a benefit of using fish oil to relieve symptoms of osteoarthritis.

Omega-3 fatty acids may also protect against atherosclerosis (hardening of the arteries), heart attack and stroke — conditions for which people with rheumatoid arthritis are at increased risk.

Fish oil is sold as a supplement in liquid, capsule or pill form. A dose of at least 3 grams a day is needed to relieve symptoms of rheumatoid arthritis. Most people can safely take 3 grams a day without adverse effects. Taking more than this amount can increase the risk of bleeding and may lower immune system response.

Other dietary sources of omega-3 fatty acids are canola oil, soybean oil, flaxseed, walnuts and wheat germ. But fish oils are high in two fatty acids, eicosapentaenoic acid (EPA) and docosahexaenoic acid (DHA), that play a role in the anti-inflammatory process.

Gamma-linolenic acid

Derived from the seeds of plants such as borage, black currant and evening primrose, gamma-linolenic acid (GLA) is an omega-6 fatty acid that can be converted in the body to compounds with anti-inflammatory properties. GLA may moderately reduce pain, joint tenderness and morning stiffness from rheumatoid arthritis.

As a dietary supplement, GLA comes in liquid or capsule form and must be taken by mouth. It can cause mild gastrointestinal side effects, such as nausea, vomiting, diarrhea and gas. The recommended dose is 1 to 2 grams daily.

Ginger

The dried or fresh root of the ginger plant may relieve joint pain and stiffness and protect the stomach from ulcers and the gastrointestinal side effects of NSAIDs. However, there's limited scientific research on this topic. A few studies have been conducted in people with osteoarthritis but not in people with rheumatoid arthritis.

Ginger is sold in several forms, including powder, extract, tincture, spice and oil. For arthritis relief, a typical dose is 1 to 2 grams of powdered ginger daily. In low doses, ginger causes few side effects. Higher doses can cause abdominal discomfort and an increased risk of bleeding and bruising. It may increase the risk of gastrointestinal bleeding from NSAIDs or corticosteroids.

Glucosamine and chondroitin

Glucosamine and chondroitin are natural compounds found in cartilage. Glucosamine derived from the outer skeletons of shellfish (chitin) is sold as a dietary supplement, often in combination with chondroitin, derived from cow and shark cartilage. Since the late 1990s, interest in glucosamine as a treatment for osteoarthritis has exploded, with sales reaching nearly $1 billion a year.

The results of more than 30 studies aren't similar enough for researchers to conclude that glucosamine improves pain and function in people with osteoarthritis of the knee. Glucosamine has shown benefits for osteoarthritis in other joints. In some instances, glucosamine appeared to reduce joint pain and tenderness as effectively as did NSAIDs and slow progression of the disease. Whether people taking glucosamine for longer periods have less joint damage compared with those taking an inactive pill (placebo) is uncertain and requires further study.

Studies also show support for the use of chondroitin in treating osteoarthritis. Like glucosamine, chondroitin appears to reduce pain and improve function in people with osteoarthritis and also may slow progressive damage.

The National Institutes of Health sponsored a carefully controlled four-year study in which glucosamine and chondroitin were used separately and together to treat more than 1,500 people with osteoarthritis of the knee. Preliminary results of the study were released in November 2005. Overall, results showed that when given separately or in combination, glucosamine and chondroitin were not more effective in treating pain than was a placebo. The study also found that the NSAID used for comparison was more effective than a placebo in relieving pain. Meanwhile, another study conducted in Europe concluded that glucosamine was more effective than acetaminophen in reducing joint pain from osteoarthritis. Glucosamine and chondroitin haven't been well studied for treating rheumatoid arthritis.

In general, glucosamine and chondroitin produce fewer adverse side effects than do NSAIDs. Glucosamine may cause mild gastrointestinal effects such as heartburn, nausea, diarrhea and constipation. If you have an allergy to shellfish, you shouldn't take glucosamine. Results of some studies in animals have suggested that glucosamine aggravates diabetes by increasing insulin resistance or decreasing insulin production, leading to elevated blood sugar levels. However, more recent research seems to refute this.

Glucosamine takes up to four weeks before it becomes most effective. Some doctors recommend starting glucosamine and an NSAID at the same time, then discontinuing the NSAID when the glucosamine begins to work.

SAM-e

S-adenosyl-methionine (SAM-e) is a dietary supplement that has gained attention as a treatment for osteoarthritis. Pronounced "SAM-ee," this compound occurs naturally in human tissues and organs. Among other functions, it helps produce and regulate hormones and cell membranes. A synthetic version of the compound is sold over-the-counter as a supplement. In Europe, SAM-e is available as a prescription medication for arthritis and depression.

SAM-e has been studied in a number of clinical trials. It appears to relieve pain from osteoarthritis as effectively as NSAIDs, with fewer side effects. It can reduce pain and improve flexibility in the knees, hips, neck, lower back and fingers. You may need to take SAM-e for up to a month before you experience significant relief from symptoms.

If side effects do occur, they may include flatulence, vomiting, diarrhea, headache and nausea. Serious problems haven't been reported in studies involving as many as 22,000 participants and lasting up to two years.

Two drawbacks of this product are its inconsistent quality and high price. Tests on SAM-e samples show that many contain little or none of the active ingredient. The butanedisulfonate salt form of SAM-e has the highest bioavailability of the ingredient.

SAM-e can have drug interactions with antidepressants, including tricyclic antidepressants and selective serotonin reuptake inhibitors (SSRIs) such as fluoxetine (Prozac), paroxetine (Paxil), sertraline (Zoloft) and others. Using SAM-e in combination with one of these drugs can cause serotonin syndrome, marked by agitation, tremors, anxiety, shivering and other symptoms. Use of tramadol (Ultram) with SAM-e also increases the risk of serotonin syndrome.

Selenium
Some studies suggest that selenium, a trace mineral with antioxidant properties, may decrease joint pain and inflammation. Other research, however, has failed to show a benefit. More research is needed before any conclusions can be drawn.

Snake venom
Snake venom has piqued the interest of both conventional and complementary and alternative medicine practitioners. The powerful effects of some snake venoms on the nervous system and their triggering of other side effects have made some researchers hopeful that these attributes can be adapted for therapeutic purposes.

Currently, no FDA-approved arthritis medications are derived from snake venom. Little scientific data supports its use in treating arthritis. Because of the toxicity of snake venom, arthritis experts warn that more research is needed to determine whether it can be used safely to play a role in the treatment of arthritis.

Superoxide dismutase (SOD)
Superoxide dismutase (SOD) is an essential enzyme found in all living cells. SOD obtained from cow liver and given as an injection was reported to relieve symptoms of osteoarthritis and rheumatoid arthritis. More research is needed, however, to establish the efficacy and safety of this product.

Thunder god vine

Traditional Chinese medicine uses extracts from a plant called thunder god vine (*Tripterygium wilfordii*) to treat several conditions, including rheumatoid arthritis. Research suggests that one or more components of the plant, including gamma-linolenic acid, may have some benefit for rheumatoid arthritis by reducing inflammation and changing the way the immune system responds to the arthritis.

Taking this herbal supplement by mouth appears to improve pain, tender and swollen joints, and physical function in people with rheumatoid arthritis. Some studies also show that thunder god vine can provide added symptom relief when used with NSAIDs or methotrexate (Rheumatrex). In addition, a topical form of thunder god vine that's spread over affected joints seems to decrease joint tenderness, swelling and stiffness.

Side effects of thunder god vine may include stomach upset, skin reactions, missed menstrual periods, vomiting, diarrhea and kidney problems. Thunder god vine can also cause reproductive problems, such as a decrease in male fertility. Many parts of this plant are toxic and may cause death if eaten.

Vitamins

Vitamins C, E and beta carotene, called antioxidants, have been studied as a possible treatment of arthritis because they may help prevent cell damage that leads to joint pain and progression of the disease. For example, the Framingham Osteoarthritis Cohort Study reported in 2004 that people with osteoarthritis who had a moderate intake (120 to 200 milligrams a day) of vitamin C had a threefold lower risk of osteoarthritis progression.

Results of studies evaluating the effectiveness of vitamin E supplements for osteoarthritis pain have been mixed. But taking vitamin E pills along with standard treatment may help reduce pain in people with rheumatoid arthritis.

Although vitamin D is best known for its bone-protecting properties, some research indicates that it might help prevent rheumatoid arthritis and osteoarthritis and may slow the progress of osteoarthritis. In addition to vitamin D pills, dietary sources of

Using supplements

If your doctor or practitioner prescribes herbal remedies, your treatment could come in one or more of several forms:

- Solids such as powders, tablets and capsules
- Teas made by pouring boiling water over fresh or dried herbs and allowing them to steep
- Liquids made by boiling herbs in water, then using the concoction to make oils or syrups
- Injections (shots)
- Creams or ointments for external use

If you decide to take an herb, read the label carefully and follow the directions. Keep track of what you take and tell your doctor. See the tips for evaluating complementary therapies found on page 194. Get as much information as you can about an herbal product or dietary supplement before trying it.

vitamin D include eggs and fortified breads, cereals and milk. Brief exposure to sunlight is the easiest way to get vitamin D.

Vitamin B-3 is made up of niacin and niacinamide. Preliminary studies suggest that niacinamide — found in meat, fish, milk, eggs, green vegetables and cereals — may be useful in the treatment of osteoarthritis. But more research is needed before a recommendation can be made about taking vitamin B-3 supplements.

Willow bark

An extract from the bark of the willow tree is widely used in Europe for musculoskeletal pain. Willow bark contains salicin, an ingredient that's chemically similar to the active ingredient in aspirin. One study of willow bark for treating osteoarthritis demonstrated possible pain-relieving qualities, but more research is needed.

Joint manipulation and massage

Manipulative and body-based methods of complementary and alternative medicine involve movement or manipulation of one or more parts of the body. Practitioners believe that manipulation can relax the tissues surrounding joints and improve circulation and joint mobility. Several methods are used.

Chiropractors use a hands-on type of adjustment called spinal manipulation. Chiropractic adjustments aim to realign your vertebrae, restore range of motion and free up your nerve pathways. Osteopathy uses manipulation to treat problems with your bones and muscles. An osteopathic doctor uses his or her hands to feel the area where you're experiencing pain. The adjustment can vary — at least 30 different types are used and may include applying pressure to the affected area or holding a body part or moving it back and forth in a precise way.

In general, the gentle stretching and massage that may accompany manipulation can be therapeutic if performed by a skilled practitioner. It's unclear, however, whether joint manipulation or spinal adjustment helps relieve joint pain from arthritis. If you have rheumatoid arthritis, avoid neck manipulations.

Many health professionals, including rheumatologists, consider massage an excellent way to ease pain and stiffness from arthritis. During a massage, a therapist uses his or her fingertips, hands and fists to knead, stroke and manipulate your body's soft tissues — your skin, muscles and tendons. Many different types of massage are available, and they're performed in a variety of settings, such as health clubs, salons, clinics and massage studios.

Massage can help stretch tight muscles, relieve muscle tension, improve flexibility, promote relaxation and reduce stress. Studies show that it can also temporarily relieve pain. If you have painful, swollen joints from rheumatoid arthritis, massage directly in that area may worsen your pain. Talk to your doctor about whether massage is an appropriate treatment for you.

Mind-body interventions

Practitioners of mind-body techniques believe that your body and mind must be in harmony to promote health. A variety of techniques are used to strengthen communication between the mind and body. These interventions enhance your mind's ability to control symptoms of illness.

Several mind-body techniques may have benefits for easing arthritis symptoms. A variety of relaxation techniques, for example, show promise for improving function and well-being in people with arthritis. Relaxation helps ease tension in your body and mind and can improve the way your body responds to stress.

Biofeedback

This relaxation method uses technology to teach you how to control certain involuntary body responses to help you manage arthritis pain.

During a biofeedback session, a therapist uses various techniques, sensors and machines to monitor and give you feedback on body functions, including heart rate, breathing patterns, body temperature and muscle activity. The feedback is intended to teach you how to lower your body temperature, slow your breathing and heart rate, and relax your muscles. This allows you to enter a relaxed state in which you can cope better with the pain. Once you learn to produce these responses in a clinical setting, you can often control them on your own, without the technology.

Some biofeedback techniques are taught in physical therapy or behavioral medicine departments in hospitals and medical centers. To find a qualified biofeedback therapist, contact the Biofeedback Certification Institute of America (BCIA) or ask your doctor or another medical practitioner with knowledge of complementary and alternative medicine for a referral.

Guided imagery

Also called visualization, guided imagery is a technique in which you use a series of relaxation methods and then call up a detailed image or images — usually very calm and peaceful in nature — that you experience with your senses. Imagining something stimulates the same parts of your brain that are affected when you actually experience what you're imagining. The message your brain receives is sent to other brain centers and to the systems in your body that regulate key functions, such as heart rate and blood pressure. This may help alleviate pain and other physical symptoms, reducing your need for pain medications.

Hypnosis

Hypnosis is an altered state of consciousness that enhances your focus and makes you more responsive to suggestions. Reaching a state of hypnosis or self-hypnosis involves training your mind to focus and then, over time, learning to achieve an increasingly deeper state of relaxation. This can help you access various levels of the mind to make positive changes.

During hypnosis, you're more open to suggestions such as being told to relax, and you become less responsive to external stimuli. Once you're trained to hypnotize yourself, you can use this technique to help manage your pain or shift your attention away from it. Several studies have found that hypnosis can be useful in pain management, although the technique hasn't been studied much specifically for arthritis.

No one's sure how hypnosis works. It appears to alter your brain wave patterns in much the same way as other relaxation techniques, influencing nerve impulses, hormones and body chemicals that affect how your brain communicates with the rest of your body.

Most but not all adults can be hypnotized. A variety of techniques exist. Learning hypnosis from a certified hypnotherapist requires motivation and patience.

Meditation

This technique helps you enter a deeply restful state that reduces your body's stress response. While there are different paths to meditation, in general, when you're meditating, you're concentrating. You can meditate by sitting quietly and focusing on your breathing or a mantra, a simple sound repeated over and over. You can also meditate while walking or jogging. By suspending the stream of thoughts that normally fill your mind, you can achieve mental calmness and relaxation.

Regular practice of meditation can slow brain waves, elevate mood and decrease muscle tension, blood pressure and heart rate.

Relaxed breathing and muscle relaxation

Learning to relax doesn't have to be difficult. Two simple techniques are relaxed breathing and progressive muscle relaxation. Try using these techniques when you feel stress, pain or muscle tension.

Stress or pain typically causes rapid, shallow breathing. This kind of breathing sustains other aspects of the body's stress response, such as rapid heart rate and perspiration. If you can get control of your breathing, the spiraling effects of acute stress will automatically become less intense. Relaxed breathing, also called diaphragmatic breathing, can help.

Follow this basic technique:

- **Inhale.** With your mouth closed and your shoulders relaxed, inhale as slowly and deeply as you can to the count of six. As you do that, push your stomach out. Allow the air to fill your diaphragm.
- **Hold.** Keep the air in your lungs as you slowly count to four.
- **Exhale.** Release the air through your mouth as you slowly count to six.
- **Repeat.** Complete the inhale-hold-exhale cycle three to five times.

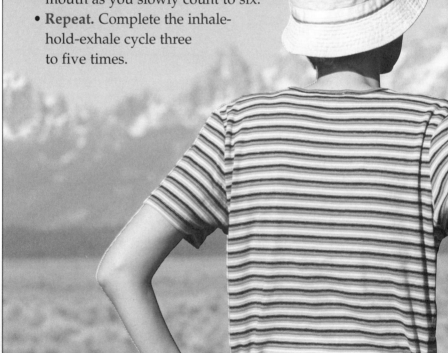

The goal of progressive muscle relaxation is to reduce the tension in your muscles. First, find a quiet place where you'll be free from interruption. Loosen tight clothing and remove your glasses or contacts if you'd like.

Tense each muscle group in your body for at least five seconds and then relax for at least 30 seconds. Repeat before moving to the next muscle group. Areas to concentrate on include face, neck, shoulders, arms, hands, chest, back, stomach, legs and feet.

As you learn to relax, you'll become more aware of muscle tension and other physical sensations caused by the stress response. Once you know what the stress response feels like, you can make a conscious effort to switch to relaxation mode. And remember, relaxation is a skill. As with any skill, your ability to relax improves with practice.

It can also lessen your body's response to the chemicals it produces when you're stressed by pain.

There are many different ways to concentrate and focus your mind. Many people start with a simple technique of sitting quietly and paying attention to their breathing. The most widely practiced form of meditation is prayer. Some types of movement, such as yoga and tai chi, can be meditative.

Prayer and spirituality

Prayer used specifically for health purposes is the most commonly used form of CAM. Surveys also show that it's one of the most widely used alternative therapies for arthritis.

People have turned to prayer and spirituality to help cope with illness and suffering for millennia. Spoken and written prayers are found in most faith traditions. Some research suggests that prayer and spiritual practice can have positive effects on health, but scientific studies haven't shown definite results of using prayer or spirituality to treat arthritis.

Although prayer alone may not "cure" your arthritis, if you find comfort, meaning and inspiration from prayer and other spiritual practices, you may be better able to cope with the effects of a chronic disease.

Yoga and tai chi

Yoga and tai chi are gentle, low-impact exercises that gradually increase strength and flexibility while also balancing mind, body and spirit to promote health and relaxation.

Yoga is a combination of breathing exercises, physical postures, meditation and other practices that originated in India more than 5,000 years ago. In the United States, many different styles of yoga are taught and practiced — one of the most common is hatha yoga, which focuses on physical poses and controlled breathing, along with meditation and relaxation.

Tai chi is a Chinese self-defense discipline that dates back at least 2,000 years. It's a self-paced series of postures or movements performed in a slow, graceful manner. Each body position flows into the next in one continuous movement.

Yoga and tai chi may relieve pain from osteoarthritis by improving strength, flexibility and balance and by helping with weight control. Studies have also shown that tai chi can improve range of motion in people with rheumatoid arthritis. Both yoga and tai chi promote relaxation and help reduce stress, which often goes hand in hand with chronic pain.

Some yoga postures can strain your lower back and joints, so be cautious and don't push to do a pose that feels uncomfortable.

Other therapies

Many other forms of CAM have been marketed for the treatment of arthritis. Among the most popular are copper bracelets, gold rings and magnets.

Copper bracelets

For decades, some people have advocated wearing copper bracelets to help fight arthritis pain. They theorize that small amounts of copper pass through your skin and neutralize free radicals — toxic molecules that damage cells.

Although wearing copper jewelry is probably harmless, most doctors find little basis on which to recommend it as a therapy for arthritis, because scientific research supporting its effectiveness is scarce. The only known side effect is discolored skin.

Gold rings

Injections of gold salts have long been prescribed to reduce inflammation and slow arthritis progression. Some researchers have speculated that the skin may be able to absorb enough gold to delay joint damage. In one small study of people with rheumatoid arthritis, those who wore a gold ring on one hand lacked deterioration in the joint nearest the ring. Joint damage caused by rheumatoid arthritis typically affects the same joint on both sides of the body.

Other research has contradicted this finding, however. Larger studies are needed to determine whether wearing a gold ring is helpful for people with arthritis.

Magnets

Some people believe that magnets can play a role in the healing process and in controlling pain. Magnets known as static or permanent magnets produce energy from magnetic fields. (Electromagnets are another type of magnet used for health purposes, usually under the supervision of a health care professional. Electromagnets generate magnetic fields only when electric current flows through them.)

Magnets are widely marketed for treatment of various diseases and conditions. They're incorporated into products such as arm and leg wraps, belts, mattress pads, shoe inserts, necklaces and other jewelry.

Researchers have investigated magnets as a possible therapy for some forms of chronic pain, including pain from arthritis. Clinical trials in this area have produced conflicting results. Some studies do suggest benefits, although it's not clear how or why magnets may work. In studies in which people do find pain relief from using magnets, the benefits are apparent very quickly.

Overall, the research to date doesn't firmly support use of magnets for pain relief. More research is needed regarding proper and effective use of the devices to recommend magnet therapy.

Words of caution

It's easy to become frustrated by the limitations of conventional medicine to treat arthritis. You may believe any possible cure is better than none. But if you opt for complementary or alternative medicine approaches, be aware of both their potential benefits and risks.

Many people turn to complementary or alternative medicine therapies because they believe they're safer or more natural than the approaches offered by conventional medicine. It's true that many conventional medical and surgical treatments have some significant side effects and health risks. But the same can be said about some CAM approaches. For example, taking the herbal remedy St. John's wort — a common treatment for mild to moderate depres-

Basics of scientific research

The randomized controlled trial is basic to most medical research designed to evaluate a new medication or other form of treatment. In this type of study, participants are randomly divided (through a computer or a table of random numbers) into two or more groups. The investigational group receives the new therapy (active treatment). The other group, called the control group, receives either the standard treatment, if there is one, or a placebo — a substance or procedure that has no known effect on the condition being studied.

In a double blind randomized controlled trial, neither the participant nor the researcher knows who received the therapy being tested. With this approach, the results are objective. Still, because of the great variability among different people, many doctors prefer to see the results of subsequent trials confirming the results of a particular study before considering the results conclusive.

sion — can dramatically alter the levels of some medications in your bloodstream, leading to one individual experiencing a heart transplant rejection. "Natural" doesn't mean the same thing as safe.

As noted throughout this chapter, evaluating the effectiveness or safety of complementary and alternative treatments can be difficult because many haven't been studied as extensively as mainstream medical practices have. The conventional form of medicine practiced by most doctors is grounded in scientific method that relies on experimentation and established research methods. Before a new treatment becomes widely accepted, scientists typically publish their results in scientific journals. These journals are reviewed by other experts who aren't associated with the experiment or the sale of the product.

Reviewers try to objectively evaluate the validity of the findings and point out any problems with the method of study or conclusions made from the results of the experimental trials. Through this process, researchers and their reviewers attempt to identify the health benefits and risks associated with a new treatment. The scientific method also attempts to distinguish effective treatments from ineffective treatments enhanced by the so-called placebo effect. This phenomenon causes some people to feel better simply because they're receiving treatment of any kind, whether it's a sugar pill or a real medication.

The cyclic nature of rheumatoid arthritis also can make it diffi-cult to gauge the effectiveness of a given treatment. Because flares and remissions can occur spontaneously (for reasons that are unclear), you may be tempted to credit relief of symptoms to what-ever treatment you recently tried. This type of "coincidental cure" can be misleading and make any treatment appear more effective than it actually is. Symptoms in osteoarthritis also can vary for rea-sons that are unclear. Changes may occur after a joint is used more strenuously than usual, or there may be no recognizable cause. Evaluation of any therapy, whether conventional or CAM, can be challenging because of these variations.

Another important fact about complementary and alternative medicine is that it's largely an unregulated industry. Unlike phar-maceutical or over-the-counter medicines, herbal preparations, vita-mins and other nutritional supplements aren't evaluated or approved by the FDA before being placed on the market. This means they can be sold without being tested for safety or effective-ness. Similarly, some complementary and alternative medicine practitioners don't need a license or other proof of competency to perform their trade.

This limited regulation also makes it easier for unscrupulous or fraudulent practitioners and businesses to prey on people who are desperate for a cure at any cost.

How to evaluate complementary medicine

The National Center for Complementary and Alternative Medicine (NCCAM) advises consumers to consider several key points before trying any complementary or alternative therapy.

- **Talk to your doctor.** Some CAM treatments can interfere with medications you may be taking or affect other health conditions you may have. You might hesitate to talk to your doctor about CAM treatments because you're afraid he or she will dismiss those options. It's true that some doctors are skeptical of CAM therapies, but as many as half the doctors in the United States refer people to CAM practitioners. Regardless of your doctor's opinion of complementary and alternative medicine, make sure you let him or her know what treatments you're using. He or she can help provide you with information about risks and benefits so that you can make informed decisions regarding these treatments.

- **Be an informed consumer.** Research what's known about the safety and effectiveness of any complementary or alternative therapy. This means finding out what scientific studies have been done and learning about the advantages and disadvantages, risks, side effects, expected results and length of treatment. You can start by asking your doctor or searching for scientific literature in your public library or university library, from NCCAM, or through medical libraries or databases on the Internet.

  You can also talk to other people with arthritis who have tried the treatment, even though they may be a less objective source of information. Remember that their testimonials can't prove how safe or effective the treatment will be for you.

- **Choose a CAM practitioner with care.** Just as you do when you choose a doctor, you'll want to examine the professional competence and experience of anyone who offers complementary or alternative treatment. If you're working with a licensed practitioner, check with your local and state medical boards for information about credentials and whether any complaints have been filed against him or her.

  If you're buying a product from a business, check with your local or state business bureau to find out whether any complaints have been filed against the company. Be wary of terms such as "quick cure," "miracle cure," "new discovery" or "secret formula." If a cure for arthritis or another disease had been discovered, it would be widely reported and prescribed or recommended. Also suspicious are claims that a product cures a wide range of unrelated diseases, such as cancer, arthritis and AIDS.

- **Estimate the total cost of the treatment.** Because many CAM approaches aren't covered by health insurance, it's essential to understand all of the costs associated with a treatment.
- **Don't substitute an unproven alternative treatment for one that has been proved effective.** Don't stop use of your medications or treatments on your own.

Make no assumptions

Complementary and alternative medicine is a fast-growing field that may offer some promising new approaches to treating arthritis. However, because the products and services are part of an industry with limited regulatory oversight, you can't assume that they're safe and effective. Become informed about the possible risks and benefits associated with a given treatment before you act. Then talk with your doctor and think it over carefully.

Chapter 8

Promising trends in diagnosis and treatment

I t's true that no one seems to be on the brink of discovering a cure for arthritis. It's also no secret that many of the treatments used to relieve the symptoms of arthritis can have limited benefits and significant side effects.

But the good news is that researchers have a clearer picture of what triggers the signs and symptoms of arthritis and causes them to continue. Although a cure isn't in sight, scientists are making significant progress in several key areas of research. As a result, the goals of treatment are moving beyond pain relief and joint preservation to prevention and reversal of damage and restoration of normal cartilage.

Several major advances have led to a better understanding of the complex interactions between certain cells and joints that lead to inflammation. Researchers are working on developing drugs and other treatments that target specific types of cells involved in the process.

The cells in your body communicate with one another using chemical messengers called cytokines (SI-toe-kines). Inhibiting or blocking cytokines that play a role in inflammation and increasing cytokines that suppress inflammation will continue to be important in developing new approaches to treating rheumatoid arthritis. Additional treatments under investigation focus on other cells that play key roles in the immune system response, such as T cells and B cells.

Targeting cytokines that contribute to the breakdown of cartilage, as well as the use of growth factors that promote healthy cartilage cells, will likely be part of the strategy for treating osteoarthritis.

In the area of surgery, treatments can repair damaged cartilage. Researchers are also exploring how gene therapy and stem cell technology may be able to restore healthy cartilage to arthritic joints.

In addition to treatments that aim to stop the disease process and restore healthy cartilage, improvements in diagnostic tools will help doctors diagnose arthritis earlier, before serious joint damage occurs.

This chapter presents an overview of some of the promising new trends and techniques in the fight against arthritis.

Improvements in diagnosis

Early diagnosis of arthritis can help prevent joint damage by allowing treatment to begin before joint tissue is destroyed. Joint damage from rheumatoid arthritis often happens within the first two years, but diagnosing the disease that early has traditionally been difficult. X-rays don't show the early changes characteristic of the disease.

One way diagnosis may be improved is by using magnetic resonance imaging (MRI) to check for cartilage loss and other changes. MRI creates high-quality pictures of both bones and soft tissues, providing a more accurate view of the entire joint. An advanced type of MRI, called dGEMRIC, detects molecules called glycosaminoglycans (GAGs), which help make strong cartilage and healthy synovial fluid. These imaging techniques allow doctors to more accurately and precisely diagnose joint problems and track responses to treatment.

Another promising diagnostic tool for arthritis is biological markers, or biomarkers — substances that can be measured in blood or urine to assess a person's risk of developing arthritis or that reflect changes in joints indicating early signs of the disease.

For example, high levels of cyclic citrullinated peptide (CCP) anti-bodies in the blood may indicate the presence of early rheumatoid arthritis (to read more about this diagnostic test, see page 47). In osteoarthritis, certain chemicals are produced as cartilage breaks down. These chemicals show promise for serving as biomarkers of osteoarthritis. In the future, tests for such substances may help diagnose the disease in its early stages.

Medications

Researchers continue to look for new medications that can more effectively prevent inflammation and joint damage, including thera-pies for patients who don't respond adequately to available drugs, and medications with less-serious side effects than those of some drugs currently in use.

The introduction of biologic agents for the treatment of rheuma-toid arthritis marked a major step forward. These drugs inhibit the cytokines interleukin-1 (IL-1) and tumor necrosis factor-alpha (TNF-alpha), both of which play a role in causing inflammation. The drugs reduce symptoms of rheumatoid arthritis, limit joint damage and improve function. Other cytokine inhibitors and new biologic agents are in development.

Agents that promote or replace cytokines that have an anti-inflammatory effect also may become available. Novel strategies of cytokine manipulation may involve gene therapy that uses DNA to prompt the body to produce beneficial cytokines and to change the balance of these chemical messengers to slow down the inflamma-tory process.

Other types of drugs, including antibiotics and estrogen, are also being investigated for use in treating arthritis. Another area of research is a vaccine to prevent the development of arthritis.

The use of new drugs in combination with currently available drugs may allow for greater control of rheumatoid and other forms of arthritis. The number of possible drug combinations increases with each new drug that's approved. (See Chapter 5 for informa-tion on treatment with established medications.)

LOX/COX inhibitors

Like nonsteroidal anti-inflammatory drugs (NSAIDs) and COX-2 inhibitors, a class of drugs called LOX/COX inhibitors block the cyclooxygenase (COX) enzyme that's involved in joint inflammation. But LOX/COX inhibitors also block the lipoxygenase (LOX) enzyme, resulting in reduction of pain and inflammation with less risk of gastrointestinal side effects such as stomach bleeding.

Licofelone is a LOX/COX inhibitor that's currently in development. Preliminary studies show that this medication is at least as effective as naproxen for treating osteoarthritis, with fewer side effects. Licofelone may also act to slow progress of the disease. Unlike traditional NSAIDs, licofelone doesn't increase the risk of stomach ulcers when taken along with low-dose aspirin. Researchers also believe that licofelone may not cause the increased risk of cardiovascular problems associated with the discontinued COX-2 inhibitors Vioxx and Bextra. Studies of the safety and effectiveness of licofelone for treatment of osteoarthritis are ongoing.

Newer types of COX-2 inhibitors are also being developed. Clinical trials are under way for lumiracoxib and etoricoxib (Arcoxia), new members of this class of drugs. But because Vioxx and other drugs of this type have been pulled from the market because of safety concerns, the Food and Drug Administration is awaiting further safety data before approving either of the new drugs. Another related class of drugs called cyclooxygenase inhibiting nitric oxide donators may improve gastrointestinal safety while providing the analgesic and anti-inflammatory effects of NSAIDS.

Biologic response modifiers

Biologic response modifiers target various parts of your body's immune system that might trigger inflammation and joint damage. TNF-alpha inhibitors (etanercept, infliximab and adalimumab) are one type of biological treatment approved for rheumatoid arthritis. Another is the interleukin-1 blocker anakinra.

New TNF inhibitors are in various stages of development. In addition, several other biologic agents are being investigated for the treatment of rheumatoid arthritis. These medications target different types of cells involved in the immune system's inflammation response.

Rituximab. Rituximab (Rituxan) reduces the number of B cells in your body. B cells produce antibodies that contribute to the development of rheumatoid arthritis. B cells also are involved in the inflammation process by activating T cells — white blood cells that play a role in switching on other cells in your immune system.

Rituximab is used to treat people with non-Hodgkin's lymphoma. In early 2006, rituximab received Food and Drug Administration (FDA) approval for use in treating rheumatoid arthritis as well, both for relieving symptoms and preventing or stopping joint damage. Studies have examined rituximab alone and in combination with other arthritis drugs, with promising results. So far rituximab has been proven safe and effective, producing significant, long-lasting improvements in rheumatoid arthritis.

Belimumab. Belimumab (LymphoStat-B) also targets B cells by blocking the activity of B lymphocyte stimulator (BLyS), a molecule that signals or activates B cells. Preliminary studies suggest that higher than normal levels of BLyS may trigger rheumatoid arthritis by stimulating production of autoantibodies, which attack the body's own healthy tissues.

In a clinical trial of belimumab, the medication reduced symptoms by at least 20 percent in more than one-third of people taking the drug. More studies are needed to confirm these results.

Tacrolimus. Tacrolimus (Prograf) is an immunosuppressant that blocks the action of T cells. Tacrolimus is approved for people who've had liver or kidney transplants. It keeps their bodies from attacking their new organs. In Japan, the medication is also approved for treating rheumatoid arthritis in people who haven't responded to other therapies. Tacrolimus may help people with rheumatoid arthritis by stopping T cells from causing inflammation.

Costimulation blockers. T cells require two signals to turn them on, and researchers hope that blocking one of those signals will render the T cells inactive, slowing the body's response to inflammation. Preliminary trials of drugs in this category, known as T cell costimulation blockers or modulators, have been conducted both alone and along with methotrexate (Rheumatrex).

In clinical trials, one of these drugs, abatacept (Orencia), effectively controlled signs and symptoms of rheumatoid arthritis.

Recently approved by the FDA, abatacept is given intravenously (IV), and side effects are generally mild. It may be used alone or in conjunction with disease-modifying antirheumatic drugs (DMARDs) other than TNF inhibitors.

Interleukin blockers. Interleukin-6 (IL-6) is a family of cytokines that are overproduced in the joints of people with rheumatoid arthritis. IL-6 is believed to be responsible for joint damage and swelling and may also be a cause of fever and excess blood platelets (thrombocytosis) in people with rheumatoid arthritis. Researchers hope that blocking IL-6 can reduce the damage it does. Early research has shown promise.

Diacerein is a drug that appears to have inhibiting effects on the production and activity of interleukins and metalloproteinases, enzymes that destroy cartilage in joints. Preliminary studies have suggested that diacerein may prevent progression of osteoarthritis, but more study is needed.

Proteasome. Proteasome is an enzyme complex that targets and interacts with a number of cellular proteins. It appears to regulate several steps of normal cell function as well as the immune reactions involved in autoimmune diseases. Blocking proteosome activity could interrupt the immune response and the release of inflammatory cytokines to reduce inflammation. At this time, however, few studies have been done to provide information about the effects of proteosome inhibition in people with these diseases.

Antibiotics

Antibiotics are traditionally used to fight infections. Scientists continue to explore the possibility that some form of infection might trigger the onset of rheumatoid arthritis. Osteoarthritis isn't believed to be caused by infection, but research has shown that antibiotics can suppress enzymes and other proteins known to cause inflammation. Researchers are exploring whether antibiotic drugs can slow or prevent joint damage that occurs in both osteoarthritis and rheumatoid arthritis.

Results from clinical trials have been mixed. Minocycline (Dynacin, Minocin, Vectrin), a tetracycline antibiotic, decreases the activity of metalloproteinases. It may provide some relief from joint

---

The promise of chemokines

The first biologic agents approved for the treatment of rheuma-toid arthritis were medications that blocked cytokines — pro-teins that influence other cells and eventually lead to inflamma-tion and joint degeneration. Now researchers are looking at a particular type of cytokine, called chemokines, as a possible next step in arthritis therapy.

Chemokines may be produced by a variety of cell types as part of the inflammatory response. Chemokines signal T cells, B cells and other immune system cells to come to the site of inflammation, such as a joint. In rheumatoid arthritis, the immune response continues in an unbalanced way, as more and more fighter cells are called to the affected joint.

There are about 50 different types of chemokines and 20 chemokine receptors, offering scientists many possible targets for interrupting the inflammatory process. Studies of chemokine-blocking agents in animals have been promising, although so far success in humans has been modest.

---

swelling, stiffness and pain in people with rheumatoid arthritis. But in some people, minocycline may actually cause arthritis symptoms.

Doxycycline (Doryx, Monodox, Periostat) is in the same family of antibiotics as minocycline and may have similar anti-inflamma-tory effects. Studies are currently being conducted to test the use of doxycycline for osteoarthritis.

Cholesterol-lowering drugs (statins)

Statin drugs such as atorvastatin (Lipitor) — widely used to lower blood cholesterol and reduce the risk of cardiovascular disease — may also have anti-inflammatory properties. In the first clinical trial to study the effect of statins on inflammation in people with rheumatoid arthritis, those who took atorvastatin had fewer swollen joints compared with people who received a placebo.

If further studies confirm these results, statin drugs may be a good option for use in combination with DMARDs. Not only would the medication help control inflammation, but it would help prevent heart disease, of which people with rheumatoid arthritis are at higher risk.

Topical medications

Researchers have tried various approaches to retain the benefits of traditional NSAIDs while avoiding the gastrointestinal problems they can cause. One solution is to put these drugs into a cream or lotion that can be applied to skin. Although no topical NSAIDs are currently approved for treating arthritis, some studies have shown a short-term benefit. For example, in a trial of a lotion containing the NSAID diclofenac, it helped ease pain and stiffness and improve function in people with osteoarthritis of the knee.

However, many studies of topical NSAIDs are short term, lasting only two to four weeks. Other research has shown that treating osteoarthritis with externally applied NSAIDs helps only for the first two weeks. After a short while, the effect is lost.

Another approach under investigation involves the use of a patch containing lidocaine (Lidoderm), a topical pain reliever. In a preliminary study involving people with knee osteoarthritis, placing the patch over the affected area produced pain relief similar to that experienced by taking celecoxib (Celebrex). More research is needed to determine the safety and effectiveness of this approach.

Hormonal and osteoporosis drugs

Because osteoarthritis becomes more prevalent in women after menopause, when levels of estrogen dwindle, doctors have long suspected that estrogen depletion may play a role in the development of the disease. Although researchers don't know why estrogen is protective, they suspect that it modifies factors involved in the natural buildup and breakdown of bone and cartilage.

Women who use oral contraceptives, which contain estrogen, have a lower risk of developing rheumatoid arthritis compared with women who don't use them. In older women, hormone therapy to supplement declining levels of estrogen has been used for years to help reduce the risk of osteoporosis. It also may offer some protection against osteoarthritis in large joints, such as the hip. In one study, women with knee osteoarthritis who took estrogen had

A different means of attack

Is controlling the growth of blood vessels a key to treating rheumatoid arthritis? Maybe.

Angiogenesis (an-jee-o-JEN-uh-sis) is the term used to describe the process of blood vessel growth. Researchers are trying to understand and better control this complex process. Most of the recent work has focused on cancer. Tumors can't grow to life-threatening size unless they're adequately nourished by blood. Therefore, they give off substances called angiogenic factors that promote the growth of tiny blood vessels.

In rheumatoid arthritis, excessive growth of blood vessels contributes to joint damage. By developing medications that control blood vessel growth, the damage may be avoided or minimized.

In the future, you may hear about anti-angiogenesis as a strategy for treating cancer, rheumatoid arthritis, psoriasis and eye diseases such as glaucoma and retinitis pigmentosa.

fewer bone abnormalities. However, research hasn't shown that estrogen replacement therapy protects women from developing rheumatoid arthritis.

Long-term use of hormone therapy is associated with health risks. For this reason, it may not be appropriate for you. Talk to your doctor about the risks and benefits of estrogen for you.

Alendronate (Fosamax) is another drug used to treat osteoporosis that may have a beneficial effect on osteoarthritis. In one study, postmenopausal women who took alendronate reported less knee pain from osteoarthritis. In addition, the women had less structural damage in their knees.

Preventive vaccines

A certain type of white blood cell, called a T cell, or T lymphocyte, is involved in initiating an immune system response that eventually leads to joint destruction in rheumatoid arthritis. Researchers are studying how a vaccine might suppress the activity of these T cells and prevent rheumatoid arthritis.

Leeches for pain relief?

It sounds positively medieval, but modern scientists are exploring the ancient practice of using leeches for medicinal purposes. In a pilot study of the use of "leech therapy" for osteoarthritis, researchers found that applying leeches to the affected knee for about an hour relieved pain, stiffness and other arthritis symptoms for at least three months.

The treatment was safe and well tolerated. More studies are necessary to confirm these preliminary findings. It's not known how it works, but perhaps some anti-inflammatory substance released from leech saliva has pain-relieving effects. The researchers hope their work may lead to the discovery of a pain reliever that could be taken without the need for a leech bite.

T cell vaccines have been tested on animals with various immune disorders. The specific types of T cell malfunction that occur in people with rheumatoid arthritis remain to be understood. In addition, vaccines that give rise to antibodies that block peptides which promote inflammation also are in the early stages of development.

Genes

Genes are the part of your chromosomes that determine your hair color, height, eye color and most other characteristics. Researchers have identified some genes that may make people more susceptible to arthritis. But a number of different genes appear to be involved, and genetic susceptibility is just one of many factors responsible for causing the disease. Still, it's important to determine how common these genetic defects are and whether they can be prevented.

Once researchers have pinpointed a problem gene or genes, they hope to develop a test to determine who's at risk of arthritis. This testing may encourage people to take steps to minimize their risks and seek medical treatment earlier. Early diagnosis and treatment are crucial tools in preventing permanent joint damage.

Gene therapy

For some diseases, gene therapy means supplying a healthy gene to the body to replace a defective gene or inserting genetic information into the defective gene to make it "healthy." In treating other diseases, gene therapy may involve blocking the action of a harmful gene or promoting the action of a helpful gene.

Specific genes may direct cells in your body to manufacture substances that help reduce inflammation, affect your body's immune responses or help protect your joints. The goal of gene therapy for arthritis is to increase production of these natural enemies of arthritis. These genes might stop inflammation of the joint lining, prevent breakdown of cartilage or stimulate growth of new cartilage cells. Two main approaches can be used. In "ex vivo" gene therapy, your own cells are removed, a specific gene sequence is inserted into them and they are returned to your body. "In vivo" gene therapy uses a vector, such as a virus that's been altered so that it doesn't cause disease, to introduce genes into your body.

Much of this research is still in the early stages. Although researchers have identified some helpful genes, they have yet to figure out the best method for delivering their protective benefits. Early studies have involved transferring genes that help preserve cartilage into the synovial lining of joints affected by osteoarthritis. These initial studies, though small, showed that the procedure can be safe and holds promise for treating the disease. Arthritis experts are hopeful that this type of treatment may have fewer side effects than do existing medications.

Gene therapy has also been used to improve results of some drug therapies. Many people with rheumatoid arthritis have had successful results from treatment with the immunosuppressant drug azathioprine (see page 106). In a small number, however, azathioprine produces life-threatening toxic reactions. Doctors at Mayo Clinic discovered a gene for thiopurine methyltransferase (TPMT) that may help predict which people are most at risk of these kinds of reactions.

Researchers found that the TPMT genes in some people have mutations that appear to cause no problems by themselves. But people with these mutant genes experience severe reactions to azathioprine. By testing patients for this mutation, doctors know when this drug can be safely prescribed.

Surgery

Advances in surgical procedures to treat arthritis are taking many directions. Joint replacement continues to improve with the development of components designed to last longer and loosen less often. The trend toward minimally invasive surgery offers hope for faster healing and quicker recovery. Computer-assisted surgery may lead to better results in the future.

Improved techniques allow surgeons to more effectively treat problem joints by removing inflamed synovial tissue (arthroscopic synovectomy). And researchers are gaining a better understanding of how the body repairs damaged cartilage. In the past several years, several methods have been advanced to repair cartilage defects.

In a technique called autologous chondrocyte implantation (ACI), cartilage cells are removed from one of your healthy joints, grown in a laboratory and then inserted into a damaged joint along with a solution that stimulates growth. Results have been promising, producing long-term improvements in joint function and decreased pain and swelling in people with osteoarthritis. Those who have been able to return to their normal activities within two years generally are able to continue these activities over the long term.

ACI typically has been used to repair small areas of damaged cartilage in the knee. More recently, the technique has been used to treat problems in the ankle, shoulder, elbow, hip and wrist. In addition, surgeons are repairing larger areas of damage. It remains to be seen whether progression of osteoarthritis will be prevented in people who've had this form of cartilage transplantation and if the procedure will prove cost-effective in the long run.

Autologous osteochondral transplantation is somewhat similar to ACI but involves the removal of plugs of bone with cartilage from non-weight-bearing sites from the same joint as the damaged one, or from the same joint on the opposite side of the body. The plugs are inserted into holes prepared in the damaged area of the joint.

Preliminary research into other forms of cartilage transplantation is also under way. A procedure called periosteal transplantation shows promise. The periosteum is a thick membrane covering the surface of bone, which is also responsible for making cartilage cells before birth. In this transplantation procedure, surgeons insert healthy periosteal cells into the damaged joint. When successful, the transplanted cells transform and start to regenerate smooth cartilage and heal the damaged joint surface. This technique may be most appropriate for younger people, since the ability of the periosteum to generate cartilage cells declines with age.

To date, among the many methods available for surgically repairing damaged cartilage, none has been able to consistently reproduce normal cartilage. No technique stands out as the optimal method. More research is needed to compare different methods and determine which produces the best long-term results. (For details on established surgical treatments, see Chapter 6.)

Future horizons

Because of the need for better treatments for arthritis, scientists continue to investigate many different avenues of potential promise. Tissue engineering is a growing field that unites cell biologists, engineers and surgeons. Tissue engineering seeks to move beyond current means of cartilage repair to the generation of new cartilage. Researchers hope to implant cartilage cells on a "scaffold" — a matrix or gel that promotes the growth of new tissue. The use of stem cells, gene therapy and cartilage growth factors (which stimulate healthy cartilage growth) may also play a role.

Stem cells are cells that give rise to other types of cells, such as bone, cartilage, muscle and immune system cells. Stem cells taken from adult bone marrow, for example, can develop into cartilage cells. Some researchers are trying to train adult stem cells from bone marrow to turn into healthy cartilage tissue as a way of regenerating damaged cartilage. This research is in the earliest stage, however, and scientists face a number of hurdles before stem cell therapy becomes practical.

Ultimately, arthritis treatment may involve an approach that combines advances in tissue engineering, gene therapy and improved medications. Treatment plans will be based on an individual's genetic background, risk factors and medical history.

Chapter 9

Tips on pain control

Sharp. Throbbing. Nagging. Stiff. Burning. Achy. Agonizing. There may be 43 million different descriptions of arthritis pain, one for each person who has arthritis. If you're like most people with arthritis, you know that no matter how you describe it, that pain could keep you from the things you would like to do today. It just won't go away. You have to deal with your pain.

Your pain is influenced by several things: your level of activity, your physical condition, the amount of swelling in your joints, your tolerance for pain and your state of mind.

Your approach to treatment may be as individual as your pain. Some approaches focus on building a lifestyle that minimizes pain. You can protect your painful joints by limiting movement and using devices to help with daily tasks (see Chapter 10). You can strengthen the muscles around damaged joints to keep them from taking the brunt of painful movements (see Chapter 11). Losing weight also may lessen the stress on painful joints (see Chapter 12). Maintaining an attitude that keeps pain in perspective is essential (see Chapter 13). The use of medication to reduce inflammation and treat pain is another part of treatment (see Chapter 5).

In many ways, this entire book is about the single most important symptom of arthritis: pain. And there are many ways to view and deal with it.

This chapter focuses on specific techniques for managing pain. The first section explains simple treatments for acute pain. Many of these can be performed at home. The second section discusses professional treatments other than medications.

Treating pain at home

Cold

For occasional flare-ups, cold may dull the sensation of pain in the first day or two. Cold has a numbing effect and decreases muscle spasms. Don't use cold treatments if you have poor circulation or numbness.

Ice packs. Before using an ice pack, apply a thin layer of mineral oil to your skin at the painful joint. Place a damp towel over the mineral oil. Finally, put the ice pack on the damp towel and cover it with several dry towels for insulation.

You may apply cold several times a day, but for no more than 15 to 20 minutes at a time. Check your skin regularly for loss of its underlying normal color. This color loss may indicate the onset of frostbite. Stop immediately if this happens.

Helpful hint: To make your own ice pack, combine ⅓ cup of rubbing alcohol with ⅔ cup of water. Place this mixture inside a freezer bag and seal it, then place the first bag inside a second, seal that and place the pack in the freezer. It's ready to use when the contents are slushy. To refreeze the contents after use, place the pack back in the freezer.

Ice massage. This method applies cold directly to your skin. Using a circular motion, move the ice in and around your painful joint for five to seven minutes. Apply mild pressure and remember to keep the ice moving when it's in contact with your skin.

Again, remember to watch for color changes in your skin. If you notice your skin losing its underlying natural tone, stop immediately. If your skin becomes numb during the massage, end the treatment early.

Helpful hint: You can make your own ice block by freezing water in a paper cup. Peel back part of the cup to expose enough ice for your massage. Wrap the cup in a small towel to protect your hands.

Heat

Heat can ease your pain, relax tense, painful muscles and increase blood flow to the affected region. But if you have poor circulation or numbness in the joint or area you plan to treat, don't apply heat. You won't know if you are getting burned. Don't apply heat after acute trauma or over a swollen area because it could increase swelling and pain.

Hot and cold packs

Perhaps the safest and most convenient commercially available product for applying either heat or cold to an affected area is the inexpensive, reusable gel-filled pack found in most pharmacies.

You typically heat the pack in hot water or a microwave oven or freeze it for application as a cold pack. The heat or cold dissipates as the pack is used, so it's generally safe to leave on for 20 to 30 minutes at a time. You can also use it to treat minor muscle sprains and strains and minor tendinitis. Be sure to follow the pack manufacturer's instructions.

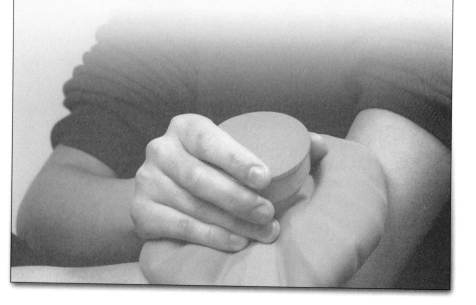

Hot packs and heating pads. Apply several layers of towels over the area to be heated with a hot pack. Lay the hot pack over the towels. Cover the hot pack with several layers of towels for insulation. Add or remove towels between your skin and the hot pack to vary the heat. You may need to add layers of towels over spots where bones project. Apply the heat for 20 to 30 minutes.

Check your skin every 15 minutes. If you see red and white blotches, stop the treatment at once. Your skin has been heated enough. Continued heating could cause a burn or blister.

To protect your skin from burning, don't lie on a hot pack or heating pad or apply pressure during treatment.

Heat lamps. Use an infrared heat lamp with a reflector heat bulb, or clamp lamps or incubator lights equipped with low-cost incandescent light bulbs. Incandescent lights release most of their energy as heat. The infrared rays produced by these types of lights cause a significant increase in local circulation in the skin and underlying tissues. Position the heat source approximately 18 to 20 inches from your skin. Apply the heat for 20 to 30 minutes. As with hot packs or heating pads, use an alarm clock or timer, or ask someone to wake you if you think you might fall asleep.

You can decrease the intensity of the heat by moving the lamp farther away. Direct the lamp at the skin from the side rather than from above.

Water: Baths, showers, whirlpools. One of the easiest and most effective ways to apply heat is to take a 15-minute hot shower or bath. You don't need an expensive hot tub. A standard bathtub can be just as effective. In a very warm bath or shower, remember to use extra caution — and the grab bars. You could become light-headed or even faint.

Contrast baths
Contrast baths are helpful to many people with rheumatoid arthritis or osteoarthritis of the hands and feet. These baths may provide more relief than hot or cold baths alone.

Start with two large pans. Fill one pan with warm water (approximately 97 to 104 F) and the other one with cool water (approximately 55 to 61 F). Place your joint in the warm water first for

The athlete

I was 26 years old when rheumatoid arthritis was diagnosed.

The news struck with shocking force. I had a husband and an infant son to care for. And I had been an athletic young woman, with high school championships in tennis and swimming. Living in Colorado, I also loved skiing throughout the long winter. In the warmer months my husband and I would bike with our friends up and over the spectacular mountain passes.

When the pain set in, it concentrated mainly in my feet and hands. Sharp pain. Dull pain. Throbbing pain. Every kind of pain you can imagine. Every step I took and every gripping action I made became horribly painful. The sensation of a single step, for instance, was akin to walking on a broken foot. The pain would begin in my joints and instantly engulf the entire foot.

My physician told me to stay as active as I possibly could. So when I was forced to give up some of my favorite pastimes, I tried to substitute others. I quit skiing but substituted snowshoeing. I gave up tennis, but became an enthusiastic hiker, walking as many as 5 miles at a stretch up and down towering mountainsides. Even with medication the pain was always there. But I learned to distract myself with thoughts: the beauty of the view, the chance to be outside in the fresh air, the sense of accomplishment I'd feel when the exercise was over.

Today, nearly all the pain is gone. The rheumatoid arthritis has been in remission for about a decade, and the osteoarthritis I got about the same time doesn't bother me. I get occasional pain in my hips, but prescribed exercises keep the joints strong and the pain at bay. My physician had said the pain might burn itself out, but I think my commitment to staying active helped a lot. I still swim a mile every day. And I've now biked in 49 states and 21 countries. In fact, even with my knee replacement five years ago, I just went on a two-week bike trip across Portugal and celebrated my 70th birthday while I was there.

Cynthia
Denver, Colo.

10 minutes and then in the cold water for one minute. Cycle back to the warm water for four minutes and then to the cold for one minute and repeat this process for half an hour. Always end with the warm water. If pans aren't handy, twin sinks work just as well.

Helpful hint: Use warm, not hot, water.

Professional help for pain

Several health care workers may be part of your pain management team: your family physician, rheumatologist, physical therapist and occupational therapist, a physiatrist, psychiatrist or psychologist, and perhaps even a practitioner of complementary medicine, such as an acupuncturist. They may use various methods and techniques to help you manage your pain.

Devices to control pain

Orthotics, which range from insoles to splints to braces, can be helpful in relieving arthritis pain.

Foot orthotics. Loss of foot or ankle support due to joint deterioration, most commonly seen in rheumatoid arthritis, can lead to strain on the accompanying knee or hip. Foot orthotics are used to help stabilize and support arthritic joints, thus reducing stress on other joints and relieving pain.

Lateral wedge inserts. These are insoles that are placed in your shoes. They may provide relief of knee pain due to osteoarthritis of the knee. It's also important to wear appropriate footwear with cushioning that properly supports your weight-bearing joints and back.

Knee braces. Braces are used on the lower limbs to decrease weight-bearing and provide stability. Knee braces are helpful to some individuals with osteoarthritis. They may help reduce pain and increase knee mobility.

Physical responses to control pain

Exercise. Exercise is perhaps your best defense against pain. A physical therapist may work with you to develop an exercise program that maximizes your range of motion and strengthens your muscles around painful joints. A complete discussion of the benefits of exercise is found in Chapter 11.

Massage. Massage can improve your circulation, help you relax, decrease local pain and reduce swelling. Some therapists are specially trained in massage techniques for people with arthritis.

If you would like to give yourself a massage or train a family member to do it, remember to stop if the massage is painful. If your joint is very swollen or painful, skip the massage of the joint and instead massage adjacent muscles. Also try a warming or cooling treatment to the joint or muscles or both. And, when giving a massage, use a lotion or massage oil to help your hands glide smoothly over the skin.

Helpful hint: If you use a massage oil or lotion, wash it off before any heat treatment to avoid burns.

Additional heat treatments. Unlike the more simplified home heat treatments, a physical therapist may use specialized techniques or equipment to provide pain relief.

Heat treatments might include soaking sore joints, particularly your hands, in a warm paraffin bath. For deep heat penetration, a physical therapist can use ultrasound or shortwave diathermy. This technique requires monitoring and can worsen some forms of arthritis. With instruction by a physical therapist, you may be able to use warm paraffin at home.

Steroid injections. Steroids reduce pain and inflammation. Your doctor may occasionally inject a cortisone drug into an acutely inflamed joint — for example, your hip, knee or ankle.

Because frequent steroid injections can accelerate joint damage, your doctor may limit the number of injections to no more than two or three each year.

Nerve block. This is an anesthetic injection that deadens the nerves to a painful area. Its use is limited because the pain relief may last only a short time.

Transcutaneous electrical nerve stimulation (TENS). For this type of nerve stimulation, electrodes are placed on your skin near the painful area. The electrodes are then attached to a small, portable, battery-powered unit. The unit generates low-level, painless electric impulses that pass through your skin to nearby

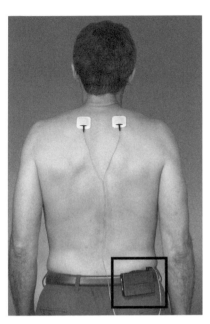

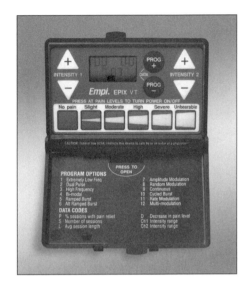

This **TENS** unit has electrodes placed for the treatment of neck pain. The lightweight unit is carried in your pocket, purse or on your belt. A control panel in the unit allows you to select the level of electric impulse.

nerve pathways in your body. You adjust settings on the TENS unit as needed to control pain.

Exactly how TENS works isn't known. It may trigger the release of endorphins — chemicals in your body that have painkilling effects similar to morphine. TENS treatment may also block nerve pathways that carry pain messages.

TENS generally works best for acute pain from a pinched nerve. This technology may be less successful for treating chronic pain, although some people with chronic pain do benefit from it. Most often, TENS is used along with exercise and other pain treatments.

A similar and newer treatment called percutaneous electronic nerve stimulation (PENS) is under study. Like TENS, this technology delivers an electric current to your nerves. But instead of transmitting the current through electrodes placed on top of your skin, PENS uses needles that penetrate your skin to just below the surface. These needles are quite thin, like those used in acupuncture. Most people feel some sensation, but not pain, when these needles are inserted.

Complementary and alternative treatments. Other treatments such as acupuncture are gaining acceptance in the medical community. A complete discussion can be found in Chapter 7.

Psychological responses to control pain

Maintaining a positive attitude is essential to coping with chronic pain (see Chapter 13). But you may reach a point at which you need some extra support or training to cope successfully. This can be an opportunity to discover a new approach to taking charge of your arthritis.

Behavior therapy. The goal of behavior therapy is to identify and modify some of your reactions to the pain, as well as to make changes to better manage your life despite your pain. This approach may include making changes in your daily routine and incorporating a balance of activities to maintain your ability to be active. You may learn to cope more effectively with changes in your lifestyle, evaluate your priorities and your response to stress, and understand and accept your pain.

Related treatments. In addition to learning behavior approaches to managing your pain, there are related treatments that can improve your functioning and may lessen your pain.

Biofeedback. Your body has some automatic reactions to stress: muscle tension, changes in skin temperature and changes in blood pressure and heart rate. The goal of biofeedback is to teach you to recognize your body's reactions to pain and learn to modify them.

During a session with a therapist, you are attached to monitors that track your physiologic systems — heart, respiration, muscle tension and skin temperature. The therapist will help you learn to reduce the symptoms of stress throughout your body through relaxation techniques.

Relaxation training. You can learn several ways to relax your body and mind. These include progressive muscle relaxation, deep breathing, guided imagery and meditation exercises.

One of the most commonly used strategies for pain is progressive muscle relaxation. You learn to focus on each muscle progressively. First, you tense a muscle and hold the tension for five to 10 seconds, focusing on the sensations of tension and identifying specific muscles or muscle groups. Then you slowly release the muscle while focusing on the sensations of relaxation and released tension. This procedure is repeated in the major muscle groups of your body so that you become familiar with the sensation of relaxing your entire body.

The ideal setting for learning relaxation is a quiet room where you can rest comfortably on the floor or in a reclining chair or bed. You need to feel relatively at ease but not tired. An instructor can be a great help in directing your attention. You will learn to concentrate and to relax at the same time — and be able to do it yourself at home. You may listen to a tape, although live training may be more effective. Eventually, you learn to relax without verbal cues from another person.

The goal of any relaxation strategy is to reduce the level of tension in your body. You can use relaxation throughout the day, when you feel tension or pain building. In this way you may prevent a worsening of the tension or pain and successfully complete your activities. For more information on deep breathing, guided imagery and meditation exercises, see Chapter 7.

Chronic pain centers. If your pain is severe, your doctor may recommend that you visit a chronic pain center. In this setting, you may undergo several days of treatment from doctors and therapists representing various specialties. Some centers require overnight stays, whereas others offer outpatient treatments.

This team approach is essential because it's unlikely that any one technique will work in controlling your pain. The professionals in an interdisciplinary center can treat both your pain and its potential consequences, such as disruption within a marriage and family, loss of income, depression and anxiety.

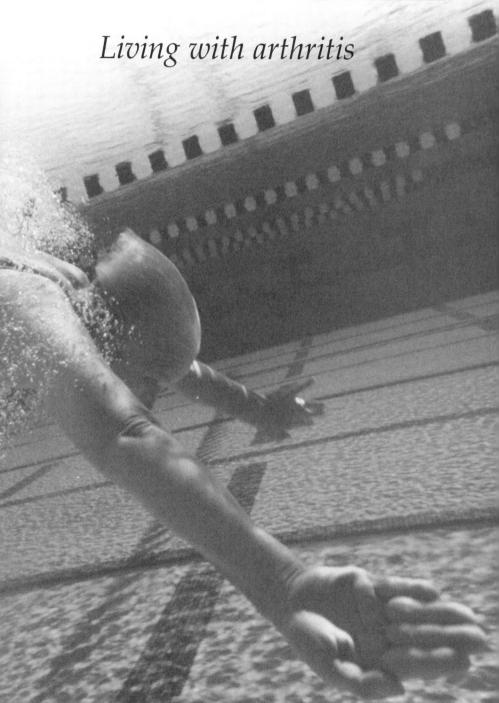

Part 3

Living with arthritis

Chapter 10

Protecting your joints

You wouldn't deliberately drive your car into a pothole or over a speed bump at 55 miles an hour. Doing either could damage your car and shorten its useful life. Neither would you go out of your way to injure your joints, especially if you have arthritis. They may be stiff and painful already, and injury would limit them — and you — even more. The goal of this chapter is to help you protect your joints from harm.

One of the most effective ways to preserve and protect your joints is to exercise. Although it might seem as if exercise will increase your risk of pain and injury, proper exercise can actually extend the life and usefulness of your joints.

Use exercise to do the following:
- Strengthen muscles surrounding your arthritic joints, providing your joints with much-needed support
- Increase your joint flexibility and range of motion
- Reduce fatigue, a major issue, especially among people with rheumatoid arthritis
- Boost your energy levels
- Help you lose weight, thereby reducing the load on your joints
- Enhance the quality of your sleep

Exercise is discussed in Chapter 11. Before you start on a physical activity plan, here are some basic principles of joint protection.

Fundamentals of joint protection

Seek medical advice

If you're not accustomed to physical activity, and especially if you're uncertain what kind of activity would be most beneficial or appropriate, check with your doctor. He or she might refer you to an occupational or physical therapist.

Warm up and cool down

You can warm up joints and muscles with a heating pad or hot pack, with massage or by gently walking in place for a few minutes. A warm bath or shower before you exercise also might help. Hot packs, applied for 20 minutes, should feel warm and soothing but not hot. Because heat could increase swelling and pain, it's important not to apply it to an already warm, swollen joint. After exercise, you may apply cold to the affected joints for 10 to 15 minutes.

Start slowly

To maintain motion without damaging your joints, move each joint through its full pain-free range of motion at least once daily. Range-of-motion exercise also provides nutrition to cartilage. The pain-free range may vary from day to day. Warm up before stretching, and take care not to overdo it, especially if you have rheumatoid arthritis.

Gently stretch muscles of affected joints at least once a day, perhaps in the morning when you get up. You may also stretch before you exercise and at the end of your exercise routine. If you have time and energy for only limited stretching, save it for after your routine. Stretching loosens your muscles and reduces the risk of injury. Slow and gentle stretching can also increase a stiff joint's range of motion. Sudden jerking or bouncing may be harmful to your joints, so aim for slow, fluid stretching motions.

Step up the pace gradually

Start at a comfortable level. That might be a walk to the end of your driveway and back. If that's what you can do, start with that. Once you're reasonably comfortable, increase the distance a little at a time.

Trim extra pounds

If you weigh more than is healthy, you have lots of company. Most Americans fall into this category. Being seriously overweight has significant implications for your health, including the condition of your joints.

If you exceed your optimal weight, you're more likely to develop osteoarthritis of the knee. And if you already have this common problem, those extra pounds can speed the breakdown of cartilage in your knee joints, leading to pain and disability. Other arthritic joints, including the back, hips, ankles, big toes and hands, can also be damaged by extra weight.

Of course, many factors may contribute to the development of arthritis. One is heredity. Another is an injury to the joint. Still another is simply the passage of time. But if you're overweight, those extra pounds can accelerate the process.

Extra pounds are also a major risk factor for diabetes and cardiovascular disease. Losing even a few pounds — a 5 percent to 10 percent weight loss — can reduce cardiovascular disease risk factors, such as high blood pressure and increased blood cholesterol, and lower your chances for knee pain and disability.

Good nutrition and proper exercise are keys to weight control. For tips on exercise and nutrition, see Chapters 11 and 12.

Try exercising at different times of the day. Find the time when you feel the least pain and stiffness.

Learn to understand and respect your pain

Learn to tell the difference between the general discomfort of arthritis and pain from overuse of a joint. Adjust your activity level or method of doing a task to avoid excessive pain. Be aware that you're more likely to damage your joints when they are painful and swollen. Don't overexercise tender, injured or badly inflamed joints.

Pain is considered excessive if it alters your breathing pattern and you find that you're holding your breath or breathing more rapidly than normal. Excessive pain is pain from which you can't

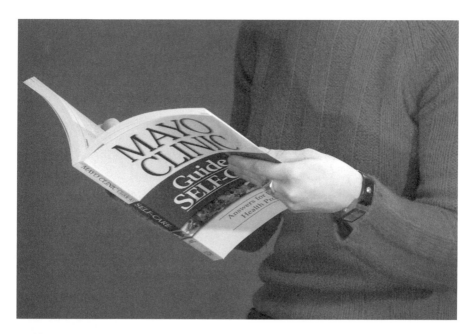

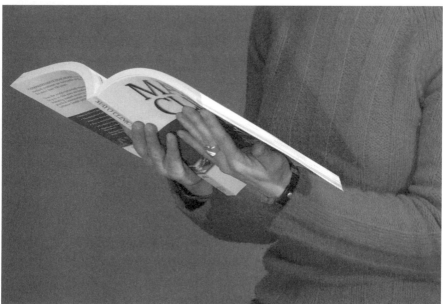

If you have arthritis in your hands, there are correct and incorrect ways to hold a book. A pinching grip (top) can strain your finger joints and may cause pain. Instead, rest the book comfortably on your palms (bottom) to ease pain.

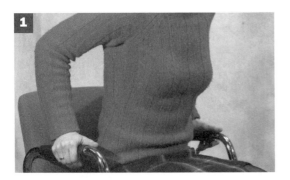

Getting up from a chair

When coming from a seated to a standing position, slide forward in the chair but don't move your feet forward. Keeping your feet slightly apart, use your legs to stand up. If necessary, push up on the arms of the chair with your palms (photo 1) or, if at a table, with your forearms (photo 2). Avoid using your knuckles (photo 3) or fingers (photo 4) to push up.

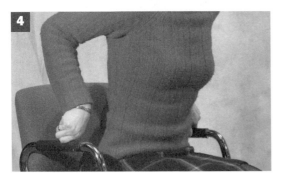

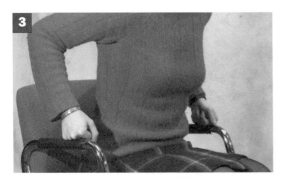

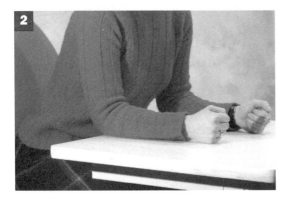

be distracted or that does not readily reduce in intensity when you stop exercising.

If increased pain lasts more than an hour or two after exercise or pain comes on more quickly day after day, chances are you're doing too much or doing inappropriate exercise.

Know your limits

If you have osteoarthritis of the hip or knee and the bones and cartilage of the affected joint aren't too worn down, then a low-impact activity such as walking might be just what you need. But if the bones and cartilage are significantly worn down, walking could cause even more damage. Non-weight-bearing activity, such as swimming or riding a stationary bike, may be a better choice.

If you have rheumatoid arthritis, non-weight-bearing activities are best, depending on the amount of wear and tear on joints affected by the arthritis. If the joint in question is not painful and a particular activity doesn't seem to cause pain, it's probably OK to proceed. But if the activity causes pain, stop and consider an alternative exercise.

Remember to rest

The concept can be confusing. First your doctor may tell you to stay active. Then you may hear about the special importance of rest.

It's a delicate balance. At times, you'll need to rest to save energy. At other times, you'll need to exercise to maintain the strength of your muscles, nourish your joints, stay reasonably flexible and build your stores of energy.

There are two forms of rest: joint rest and whole-body rest. It's important to obtain both.

Joint rest. When joints are injured or badly inflamed, they need to rest and may require immobilization with splints. The joints may be gradually mobilized when the acute problem is resolved. Using an affected joint helps keep it healthy and promotes the supply of nutrients and oxygen to the joint. Even so, individual joints can become fatigued after periods of exertion. So if your hip muscles seem tired during the day, that's a good signal to sit down and rest.

Whole-body rest. If you have arthritis, and especially if you have rheumatoid arthritis, a well-rested body is an important goal to achieve on a daily basis. Your rheumatoid arthritis makes you especially vulnerable to fatigue because many of your joints may be inflamed. In addition, inflammation may be present in organs of your body. Your condition can also cause anemia, which contributes to your fatigue.

Fatigue associated with arthritis is a deep-down exhaustion, often including muscle weakness. It can make virtually everything you attempt to do seem like too great an effort. It can leave you feeling almost helpless. You may begin to wonder if you have any control over your life.

The process of inflammation can cause pain that may bring on fatigue. If you experience a period of joint inflammation (flare), you need to schedule more time to rest your joints throughout the day. Joint pain might also cause you to change positions periodically to take weight off the affected joints. Pain can also cause you to lose sleep or prevent you from sleeping well.

If you're exhausted, you may not feel like doing much. But if you don't engage in enough physical activity, your muscles will only get weaker, and you'll find it even more difficult to get started with physical activity.

Alternatively, maybe you tend to keep on working until a job is done, regardless of discomfort — whether walking to the corner and back or finishing the laundry. That strategy might not be the best either. If you exercise too strenuously or too often without taking a break, you can strain muscles and joints and risk injury.

The key is to rest before you become too tired. Pace yourself. Don't work through those tired periods. Divide exercise or work activities into short segments with frequent breaks. Plan 10 minutes of rest every hour during periods of physical exertion. On the surface, that approach may sound disruptive and unreasonable, but it works.

From time to time during each day, find a comfortable position and relax for a while. An easy chair, a couch, a bed or a reclined seat in your parked vehicle are all potential options. You don't need to sleep, but you do need to give your body a break.

When it's bedtime, go to bed. Avoid the temptations of watching the late news on TV or finishing a book chapter. A good night's sleep will give your joints the rest they need. It can also help restore your energy and enable you to deal more effectively with pain.

If you have rheumatoid arthritis, set a goal of eight or nine hours of sleep each night. If you have trouble sleeping, talk to your doctor about it promptly. When sleep disturbances are treated, fatigue usually improves.

Using assistive devices

Observing the basic principles of joint protection can help you extend the life of your joints. But even if you do your best to preserve your joints and reduce wear and tear, the basic measures may be insufficient. A painful knee may need a brace for support. Or you might opt for a cane to take weight off the joint as you walk. If your hands are affected, various helpful tools and gadgets are readily available to help you maintain your lifestyle.

People sometimes avoid assistive devices, believing they don't need the help or thinking that the use of special measures is a form of surrender. Some people believe an assistive device such as a cane will make them look old or may lead to loss of function. In reality, assistive devices allow you to be more independent with tasks and, in so doing, play an important role in self-management of arthritis.

Think about this: Few people think twice about getting into an automobile for a drive across town. But a car, in reality, is an assistive device. It makes it easier to accomplish a goal — in this case, to get from one place to another quicker and more comfortably.

Assistive devices do much the same thing. They're a means to an end. They make it easier for you to perform everyday activities, such as opening a stubborn jar or taking a shower.

Medical supply houses and catalogs offer various items. Most of them are inexpensive and affordable. For a list of resources, see Chapter 16.

Sometimes, a little creativity is all you need. You can use plastic foam tubing, the kind used to insulate plumbing pipes in homes, to

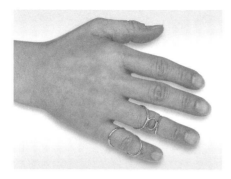 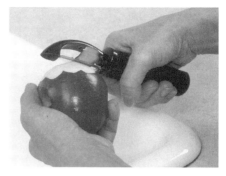

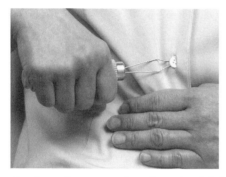 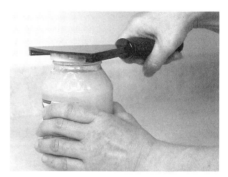

Devices to support and protect joints

Clockwise from top left: Silver ring splints limit how far you can move your finger joints. They're less cumbersome than a traditional splint, so you can wear several on the same hand. A peeler with a thick rubber handle minimizes gripping action. A specially designed jar opener reduces twisting force to a slight turn. A thin wire hook helps you grasp a button and pull it through the buttonhole.

make tools and utensils easier to grasp. The insulation is available in different sizes and can be cut to fit all kinds of hand-held devices. The foam insulation also reduces vibration.

Selection of the right assistive device can minimize joint stress. Here are tips on using some of the many options available to you:

Hand aids

Look for aids that offer a wide-diameter grip. Most toothbrushes, for example, have thin handles that force you to grasp them with a tightly closed fist. If you have arthritis, this position can put painful stress on the joints and other structures of your fingers, thumb and wrist.

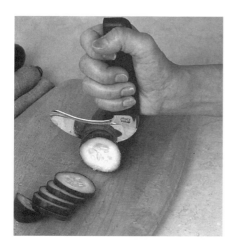

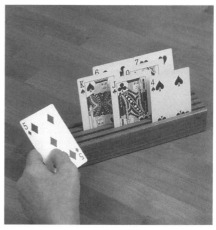

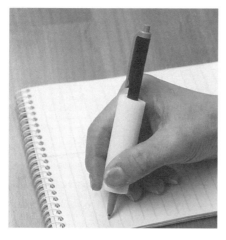

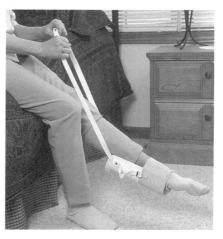

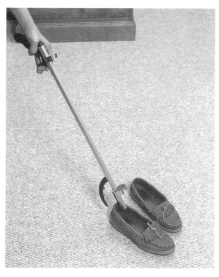

Handy household helpers

Inexpensive assistive devices are widely available. A special kitchen knife (top left), a convenient holder for playing cards (top right), a plastic foam writing grip that can help you better grasp a pen or pencil (middle left), a stocking aid that enables you to put on socks or stockings without bending down (middle right) and a "reacher" for picking up items (bottom left).

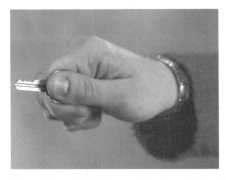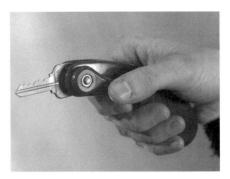

If you have arthritis in your hands, avoid making a tight fist or pinching objects tightly.
Instead, use a grasp that places your knuckles parallel to the handle of the tool or utensil.
Consider using a special key holder (above right) to help you turn keys more comfortably.

If you have arthritis in your hands, avoid making a tight fist or tightly pinching an object. A less physically stressful position is one in which your fingers and thumb aren't tightly closed.

Grooming and personal hygiene
If you have limited range of motion, you might want to opt for long-handled brushes and combs. Bathing aids such as long-handled sponges and brushes can help you reach your feet and other parts of your body with less effort and pain. Use an electric toothbrush, a toothbrush with a specially designed handle or one with a foam handle (see photo on next page). Use mirrors with foam rubber handles for an easier grasp. Bath benches, grab bars and toilet seat risers (see photo on next page) can help you bathe and take care of your personal hygiene with greater ease, safety and independence.

Getting dressed
If you have trouble reaching your feet, buy a shoehorn with an extension handle. Shop around for a stocking aid that enables you to pull on hosiery without having to bend over. Look for tools that grip buttons and zippers. Sew elasticized Velcro tabs onto shirt cuffs to allow the cuff to stretch as you slip your hand through, or sew cuff buttons on with elasticized thread.

Select wraparound skirts or stretch trousers if you have limited range of motion and dressing is a challenge. Clip-on neckties are

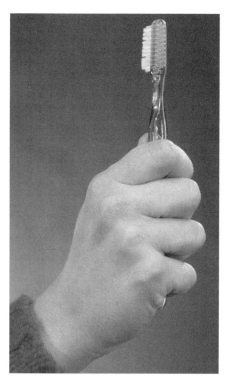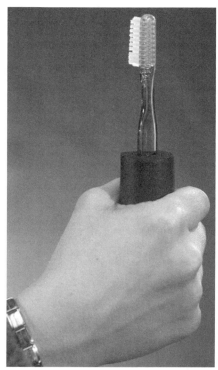

A foam tube that slides onto objects such as a toothbrush can make them easier to grip.

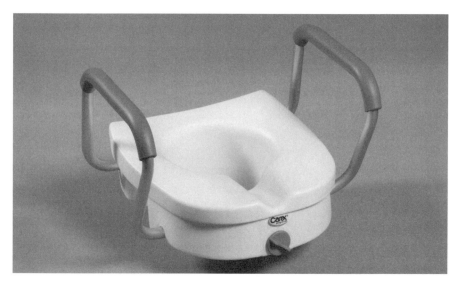

If arthritis in your hips or knees makes it difficult for you to sit down and stand up, a raised toilet seat such as the one shown above may help. It attaches directly to the toilet.

Be kind to your joints every day

An important part of joint protection is simply avoiding situations that aggravate your condition. But how do you put that advice into practice in your daily life? Try these tips:

- When writing, use good posture and lighting. Relax your hand and neck often. If holding a pen is painful, use a larger or built-up pen. Nylon-tip or rolling-ball pens require less pressure than pencils and ballpoint pens.
- Install lever-type door handles instead of knobs on doors in your home.
- Use a utility cart to transport heavy items and to avoid extra trips when moving lawn supplies, unloading groceries and performing other tasks around the house.
- When traveling with luggage, use a lightweight cart with wheels, or buy luggage with built-in wheels.
- During any activity, sit instead of stand whenever possible.

convenient, or with a regular necktie, leave the knot tied and slip the tie over your head.

In the kitchen

Organize your work area. Make sure everything you use often is easy to reach. Store frequently used cookware and utensils in cabinets at hip-to-shoulder height. Eliminate things you seldom use.

A single-lever faucet in your kitchen sink can make the numerous tasks you perform at the sink a little less taxing on your finger joints.

An electric can opener is easier to operate than a manual opener. The same is true for carving knives. An electric knife can make some kitchen work go more smoothly. Buy a cutting board that features tiny raised spikes to hold foods firmly in place while you cut them. If you use a nonelectric knife, buy one that's L-shaped with a wide-diameter vertical handle. To use this type of knife, grasp it like a dagger and use a sawing motion without applying much pressure.

In the grocery store, select prepared foods that don't require slicing and dicing. Chopped nuts, for example, cost a little more but save you time and effort. Buy a jar opener that can be mounted under a kitchen cabinet or counter.

Cleaning your home

For housework, use a long-handled mop, dustpan and broom. A sponge can enable you to use an open hand when washing windows. Store cleaning supplies on each floor and within easy reach.

If you have a front-loading clothes washer or dryer, consider placing it on wooden blocks for easier access. Avoid unnecessary bending or stooping.

Using straps

Try looping a strap through the door handle of your refrigerator if you have a hard time opening the door with your hand. Pass your arm through the strap and pull the door open. Use a briefcase with a shoulder strap to help avoid carrying heavy objects with your hands.

In the shop

For some activities, there's no alternative for a manual tool. But in many cases, there's a powered alternative. For example, a power nail driver may be easier to use than a hammer. A power screwdriver likely will be easier on your joints than a conventional screwdriver. In addition, buy lightweight tools when appropriate.

Using a brace

Along with devices designed for specific chores, you might need to give a painful joint external support with a brace. Any brace, and especially a knee brace, should fit properly. It's important to work with your doctor and physical therapist to get a good fit.

Think of a brace as a splint you can remove. Pain and swelling can be helped by immobilizing a joint. Depending on the type of brace, it may offer a long-term solution to the problem of pain.

Using a cane

A cane that's fitted to your body can provide welcome support and increase your independence. A poorly fitted cane, however, may increase your problems.

It's a common mistake to choose a cane that's too long. This pushes one side of your body up, putting strain on your shoulder joint and arm muscles. And a cane that's too short causes you to lean forward, putting extra pressure on nerves in your wrist. Whether too long or too short, a cane that's not fitted properly may throw you off balance and make you less stable on your feet.

When buying a cane, don't base your decision on looks alone. A distinctive cane may add flair to your appearance, but there are more important factors to consider:

Select the right style. If you plan to use your cane daily, the traditional candy-cane style — with curved handle — probably isn't the best choice, especially if you have arthritis in your hands. This cane doesn't center your weight over the staff, which puts pressure on your hand. Instead, consider a swan-neck cane or one with a grip that straddles the pole part of the cane. In addition, a lightweight cane is less of a burden than a heavy one. If you have severe arthritis in your hand, a platform attachment that distributes the pressure over your entire forearm may be more comfortable.

Consider length. To determine the proper length, stand erect with your shoes on. Hold your arms at your sides. The length of the cane should equal the distance from the crease in your wrist to the floor.

When you hold your cane while standing still, your elbow should flex 20 to 30 degrees. Remember, if you plan to use the cane alternately with shoe heels of varying heights, make sure you get an adjustable cane. Nonadjustable canes can be cut to fit, but then the shoes you wear must all have the same heel height.

Get a good grip. A handle with a large diameter is generally easier to hold for extended periods. Make sure your fingers and thumb don't overlap when you grip the handle. If you have arthritis in your hands, ask your doctor or physical therapist to advise you about grip size.

Check the tip. Your cane should have a removable rubber tip, 1 to 2 inches wide, for good traction and safety. Check the tip regularly. Replace it before it wears down and becomes smooth.

For cold climates, you can get an attachable steel spike for times when you find yourself on a patch of ice.

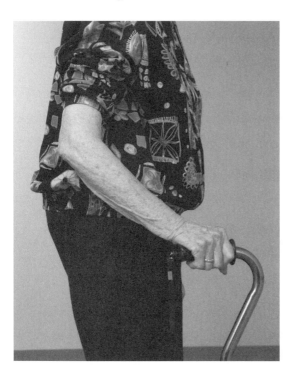

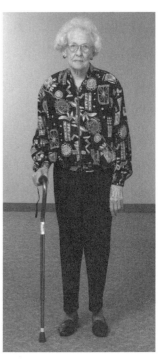

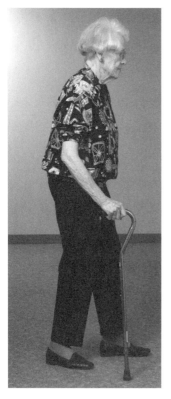

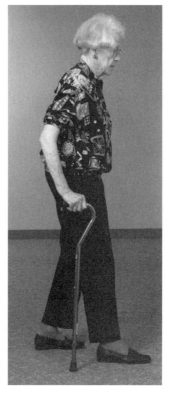

It's important that a cane fits properly. With the cane in your hand, the bend in your elbow should be about a 30-degree angle (top left). If you have a disability affecting one of your legs, grip the cane in the hand opposite the affected leg. Move the cane in unison with your affected leg (bottom left and right).

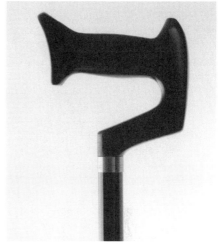

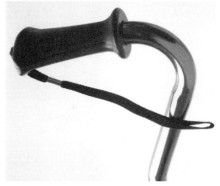

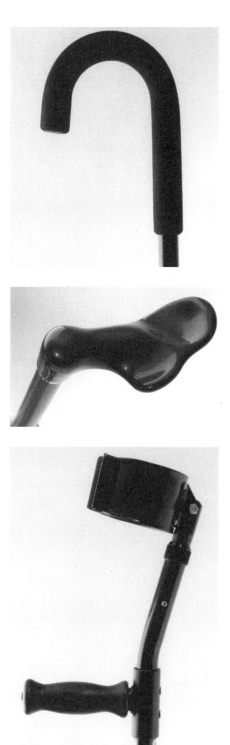

When selecting a cane, choose a grip that feels good in your hand. You might prefer a cane with a foam grip or a grip that's shaped to fit your hand. Choosing a grip is a matter of personal preference, though if you have difficulty using your fingers or your hand is injured, your doctor or physical therapist may recommend a specialized type of grip for you.

Numbness or pain in your hand or fingers may signal that your cane's grip isn't a good fit. Try out various grips before selecting one.

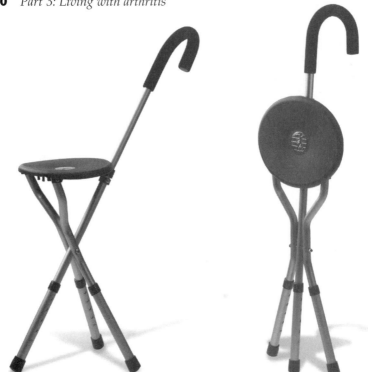

Canes come in many styles, including some that include a folding seat. Such canes can come in handy when you're doing a lot of walking and periodically need to sit and rest.

You'll get the most from your cane if you hold it on the side opposite your weaker or painful hip, knee or leg and move your weaker leg and the cane at the same time. This improves your balance and stability and takes stress off the painful or weaker side.

Put as much weight on your cane as necessary to make walking comfortable, stable and smooth. When you go up stairs, lead with the cane and your "good" foot. Then follow with the "bad" foot. When you go down stairs, do the opposite. Either way, use the railing with your free hand.

Once you've obtained a cane that fits and you've used it for a while, decide if it's a help or hindrance. If you've recovered from joint replacement surgery, retire your cane.

If you're receiving Medicare and your doctor writes a prescription for a cane, Medicare will share the cost. Most health insurance companies also provide coverage. But be sure to ask your physician to write "needed for walking" on the prescription.

Chapter 11

Exercising properly

Keep moving. That's good advice, whether you have arthritis or not. This chapter discusses the benefits of exercise and helps you assess your fitness level and set goals. It also provides you with information and specific exercises to get started. Even so, it's important to remember that you're the expert. You alone know how you feel. Only you — with the benefit of experience — can know how much is too much. Your exercise program will become increasingly effective as you listen to your body and act accordingly.

Importance of exercise

For most of us, regular physical activity is essential to health. Aerobic exercise contributes greatly to cardiovascular fitness. Cardiovascular health is more complex than how efficiently your heart pumps and how well you breathe. It involves how well your muscles and tissues absorb oxygen from your blood. It includes the density of the small blood vessels (capillaries) that feed your tissues. Body composition also affects cardiovascular health. So does your body's ability to process fat or fat-like substances (lipids) found in your blood. Prolonged bed rest or inactivity can interfere with these functions and lead to decreased cardiovascular health. Physical inactivity causes reduced circulation in your legs. It also decreases your body's ability to use oxygen. Lack of exercise can lead to loss of bone density and cause your muscles to become weakened and lose flexibility. It may also contribute to feelings of dependency, discouragement and depression.

Exercise is part of the solution for the most common complaints of people with arthritis. Most people with arthritis say their No. 1 problem is pain. Appropriate types and amounts of exercise help reduce the pain that arthritis causes. The second most common complaint of people with arthritis is fatigue. The prescription for addressing fatigue is adequate rest and aerobic conditioning.

Years ago doctors recommended rest, joint protection and medication for people with arthritis — still an important part of good advice during flares. But a healthy balance between suitable exercise and rest is important. "Let comfort be your guide" is a good rule to follow. But be careful about skipping your exercise. It takes at least three days to come back from the fitness you lose during each day of inactivity. If a flare is preventing you from taking your usual 45-minute walk, try to accumulate the 45 minutes in smaller segments. If it's painful to walk on a hard surface, try riding a bicycle or walking in a swimming pool. In addition, don't stop other parts of your fitness program. For example, continue your flexibility exercises.

A sensible exercise program can reduce your risk of cardiovascular disease and increase your endurance. It can help slow bone loss that leads to a thinning of your bones (osteoporosis), which makes them prone to breaking. Appropriate exercise increases flexibility and strengthens the muscles that help stabilize your joints. It helps reduce morning stiffness and maintain mobility. It improves your balance and increases your endurance. And, especially important for people with arthritis, exercise can help you control your weight. This helps you avoid placing unnecessary stress on your joints. Exercise makes it easier to carry grocery bags, step in and out of the bathtub, get in and out of your car and avoid falls. In addition to these physical benefits, exercise boosts you psychologically and gives you a renewed sense of well-being. It's a fact that people with arthritis who are fit fare better than those who aren't.

Tailoring your program

A one-size-fits-all approach to exercise doesn't work for people with arthritis. The only expert on the subject of you is you. Learn to pay attention to your body. Experience is the best teacher of what level of activity is appropriate for you. Remember how you feel as you begin an activity. When you're finished, note again how you feel. Are you the same or better? How about two hours — or two days — later? An activity level that's appropriate for you should make you feel the same or better afterward. If you feel worse, especially after several hours or the next day, there's something wrong with what you're doing. You may be overdoing it. Or you may be performing an activity in a way that aggravates your condition. When your body talks — listen. Don't repeat the same activity in the same way and at the same level the next day. Build up gradually or ask a physical therapist or your doctor to help you determine whether you're doing the activity most effectively.

Before you begin or change your exercise routine, have a thorough physical examination and discuss your plans with your doctor. It helps if your doctor knows about your specific needs. Talk about whether you should consult with a physical therapist or an occupational therapist. These individuals are trained to help people find ways to move effectively. A therapist who has been successful working with people who have arthritis may often be very helpful. But here again, remember that you are the expert. A therapist — or even a doctor — can't know how you feel as well as you can.

A program that's well designed should include activities you enjoy. Some people enjoy exercising with family members or friends. Walking is a good way to start. Again, your goals can be very different from those of someone else with arthritis. And, as you listen to your body, your goals can change from day to day as your condition changes.

Some people with arthritis are glad when they can walk a step or two. Perhaps you can easily walk several miles. In either case, walking is an excellent activity for overall conditioning. It improves cardiovascular health and bone density. Walking also helps your muscles and joints get nourishment. It leads to improved flexibility, strength and balance, which can help keep stumbles from becoming falls. If you don't enjoy walking, you may prefer swimming, water aerobics, biking or cross-country skiing, either outdoors or on stationary machines indoors. These fitness activities help you manage your normal daily activities without becoming winded or dizzy, breaking into a sweat or experiencing fatigue. They also help you control your weight and sleep better.

Include activities daily to improve flexibility. Stretching and range-of-motion exercises counteract the stiffness that arthritis causes in your major joints and spine. Muscles that have a high level of elasticity are less susceptible to injury. Again, a doctor or physical therapist can tell you the proper way to stretch a muscle, but only you know when it's stretched too far or for too long. Moderate, regular exercise is the emphasis of guidelines from the Centers for Disease Control and Prevention, the American Heart Association, the American College of Sports Medicine and others. The frequency and duration of activity are more important than the intensity.

Your activity goals

Guidelines recommend at least 30 minutes of moderately intense physical activity most days. Be creative about including exercise in your lifestyle. Watch TV while you're on a treadmill. Read a magazine or book while you ride a stationary bicycle. Schedule exercise into your day as you would a round of golf. Although sustained, continuous exercise may give the greatest benefit, you don't need to do all of your exercise at one time during the day. You also benefit from short periods of activity, perhaps in five- to 10-minute intervals, that add up to at least 30 minutes. The key is the total amount of energy expended, not the intensity. If you can't carry on a conversation or if you experience moderate pain while you exercise, you're pushing too hard. Walking with family or friends can be a way to combine exercise with quality time together. Walking with children provides them with a role model for lifetime habits of healthy activity.

Every move counts

Normal daily activities, as well as formal exercise sessions, add up. You get health benefits from carrying out the trash, cleaning, shopping, vacuuming, making the bed and mowing the lawn. But consider these activities a supplement to, not a substitute for, your regular exercises. And don't forget to balance these tasks with rest.

You can boost your exercise total by increasing physical activity in your routine daily tasks. Park your car farther away from your destination and walk a little farther. Or walk your dog farther than around the block.

A word of warning: Remember that body mechanics and positioning during exercise are very important. Poor positioning or body mechanics can make joints more painful or cause swelling. Some positions may be stressful to certain joints. For example, if you can't find a comfortable position for vacuuming, ask a physical therapist to help you find a comfortable position.

High-impact activities, such as jogging, basketball and some aerobics classes, put stress on your joints and may aggravate your symptoms. Substitute low-intensity activities, such as walking, low-impact social dancing or gentle water exercise. If you are able, use moderately intense activities, such as brisk walking, swimming, water aerobics, bicycling, cross-country skiing, low-impact aerobic dancing or rowing.

Organized programs

Some people enjoy participating in one or more of the numerous exercise programs that address special needs of people with arthritis. Your doctor or physical therapist can provide information about whether these routines may suit your needs. Many routines focus on simple chair exercises and arm and leg movements, using light weights and frequent repetitions for upper and lower body conditioning. Be careful with frequent repetition, especially if you have rheumatoid arthritis, because it can aggravate joint pain. Chair exercises don't help maintain bone strength as well as weight-bearing exercises do. If you're able, add walking to such a routine. When gauging an exercise program, take into consideration your other daily activities. Make sure you don't exercise a joint or muscle group too much. Activities you may wish to consider include those listed here.

Water exercise. Water exercises are especially beneficial. Soothing, warm water (between 83 and 88 F) relaxes your muscles. Your buoyancy in water relieves stress on joints, and the water offers muscle-strengthening resistance.

Tai chi (TIE-chee). People use the ancient Chinese martial art of tai chi to relax and strengthen muscles and joints and reduce tension in the body and mind. Tai chi's slow, deliberate circular movements and postures combined with deep, regular breathing can increase circulation, relax the mind and body and ease chronic pain.

Videos. Numerous exercise videos are designed specifically for people with arthritis. Some videos may contain movements not appropriate for your level of strength or ability. Discuss each exercise on the video with your physical therapist. Discontinue movements that seem too difficult, cause pain or cause joint swelling.

The Arthritis Foundation has developed a video titled People with Arthritis Can Exercise (PACE). Level 1 offers gentle routines that include stretching, strengthening and fitness exercises, and Level 2 is a moderate program designed to increase range of motion and endurance.

Assess your fitness

Fitness has many components, including aerobic capacity, muscular fitness, appropriate body composition and good posture. Earlier in this chapter, the discussion on cardiovascular fitness described the benefits of aerobic exercise. Walking, biking, swimming and cross-country skiing are good aerobic exercises for people with arthritis.

Muscular fitness is a general term. It includes flexibility, range of motion, endurance and strength. Range of motion refers to how far

Tai chi for chronic pain

Tai chi was developed more than 1,000 years ago. Literally hundreds of combinations of movement are involved in tai chi. But the focus of the exercise remains consistent, and it includes concentration, stretching, balance and grace. Doing tai chi daily can increase range of motion and strengthen muscles for a combined mind and body workout.

Although there are several schools of thought for learning tai chi, all focus on these essentials:

- **Your body is relaxed.** Motion is even and fluid. Your body is balanced and steady. Muscles aren't rigid, and breathing is deep and steady.
- **Your mind is tranquil but alert.** You concentrate on movement.
- **Your body movements are coordinated.** Hands, eyes, trunk and limbs perform as a whole. Movements are gentle, and you're constantly moving.

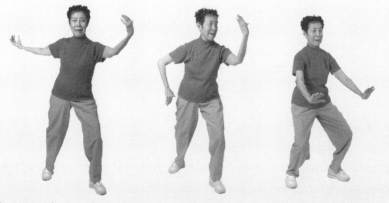

These exercises are just part of one group of tai chi movements. You do all the movements within the group as one fluid motion.

and in what direction a joint will move. It also measures a muscle's capacity to stretch. If your muscles can't stretch far enough, your joint may be fine, but its range of motion will be limited. Stretches are good for improving flexibility. But they may be challenging and painful if you have severe osteoarthritis or rheumatoid arthritis. It's easy to hurt yourself by stretching too much.

If you have arthritis, activities designed for specific strengthening often are very challenging. Before adding strengthening exercises to your program, consult a physical therapist experienced in working with people who have arthritis. You should receive careful instruction. Review your progress with the therapist periodically. You're less likely to hurt yourself and more likely to enjoy exercise if you begin an exercise program with walking and range-of-motion activities.

Body composition refers to the proportions of bone, muscle and fat in your body. Are you lean and muscular or overweight? Inappropriate body composition contributes to the pain of arthritis. Osteoarthritis also worsens if you're overweight. Having excess pounds to carry around increases fatigue. For help determining whether you're overweight, use the body mass index chart on page 266 to find your BMI. A BMI of 25 or greater means you're overweight. For people who are overweight, reasonable weight loss can increase energy and endurance.

Good posture is important for everyone. But it's especially important when you have arthritis. Many people with arthritis have increased pain as a result of poor posture. If you're not physically fit, your body may tend to sag. Lack of endurance and good muscle tone can reduce your ability to hold your body in good posture. The solution to posture problems isn't as simple as your mother's direction to "straighten up."

Good posture doesn't mean holding yourself in a rigid or sway-backed position. Normally, a person with good posture shifts constantly. Movement brings nutrition to your cartilage and joint surfaces. In fact, the wiggling movements of a 5-year-old are very conducive to good posture, but sitting all day is not. The easiest way to improve your posture is through walking. The faster you walk, the harder your muscles must work to keep you upright and straight. Some people find that swimming also helps improve their posture.

The following self-assessment tests may help you judge your current fitness level. If the activities described are too strenuous, ask your doctor or physical therapist for an appropriate substitute. Before you do any of these activities, warm up the muscles used for that activity by stretching them gently or do range-of-motion exercises. Start an exercise journal. Make notes to use as benchmarks in tracking your progress.

Aerobic fitness
Take a walking test for a distance you can manage, whether it's 10 feet or a mile. Find a place where you can walk on a level surface. Note the time on your watch and begin walking at a comfortable pace. Walk as briskly as you comfortably can. If you're too winded to carry on a conversation, you're walking too fast. After you walk the distance you've determined, check your watch and record your time.

Muscular fitness
- To check your upper body strength, do push-ups. Do this cautiously, or substitute another activity if your arthritis affects your hands, wrists, elbows or shoulders. Stand an arm's length from a wall with your palms flat on the wall. Lean into the wall, then push away. Repeat. Stop when you need to rest and record how many push-ups you did.
- To check your balance, stand near a wall (in case you begin to fall). Record how long you can stand on each foot alone.
- To measure your hamstring flexibility and strength, sit in a chair. Straighten your legs as far as you can in front of you. Measure the distance of your heel from the floor or notice the angle of your knee. Be careful not to hurt your back.
- With one hand at a time, reach behind you and as far as you can across your back.

Posture
- Observe and note your body posture as you stand facing a full-length mirror. Your ear should be in line with your instep. Your lower spine will curve in slightly.
- Stand upright with your heels next to the wall, resting your buttocks, back and head on the wall. You should have a space to fit your arm between your lower back and the wall.
- Sit in a chair with your buttocks at the back of the chair and your feet resting flat on the floor. Your thighs should be parallel to the floor.

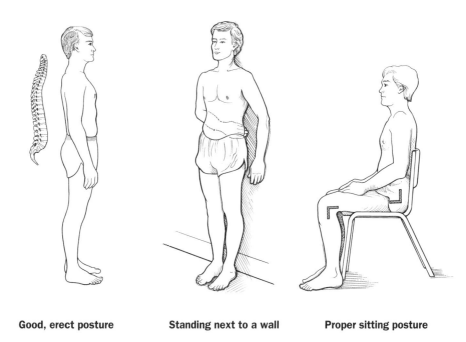

Good, erect posture   Standing next to a wall   Proper sitting posture

Getting started

Generally speaking, exercise whenever it's best for you. Try to loosen up with exercises first thing in the morning. Keep in mind that exercising at least five to six hours before bedtime may help you sleep better and feel less stiff in the morning.

Avoid exercising right after you eat. Move with a slow, steady rhythm. Don't jerk or bounce. Maintain good posture while you exercise.

Avoid exercising tender, injured or severely inflamed joints. If you feel new joint pain, stop. New pain that lasts for two hours or more after you exercise probably means you've overdone it. Rest and take an over-the-counter pain reliever as needed. Next time, break the activity into smaller segments or reduce the intensity or number of repetitions. If pain persists for more than a few days, call your doctor. With some creativity, you can continue gentle exercises during a flare, unless you have a fractured bone. If a flare in your knee limits your walking distance, try a cane, walk in a swimming pool or use a stationary bicycle set with no resistance.

Warm up your muscles with a warm shower or bath, heat packs or massage before exercising. But don't apply heat to an already inflamed joint. After exercise it may help to apply either heat or cold to affected joints for 10 to 15 minutes. If you're not regularly taking an anti-inflammatory medication and if heat and cold don't relieve your pain, aspirin, another nonsteroidal anti-inflammatory drug or acetaminophen taken an hour before exercise may limit swelling and reduce pain. Avoid mixing medications, and avoid overmedicating because you may mask pain that warns you to stop. If you already treat your pain with daily medication and can't exercise without pain, you may need the help of a physical therapist. Don't force an exercise or motion. Start gradually. You may feel slight discomfort but shouldn't feel new pain. Try doing a little less each time but add a few more sessions during the day.

Always allow time to warm up with gentle range-of-motion exercises. Gently stretch your hamstring muscles (see page 260) or begin walking slowly. Start flexibility exercises (see page 253). At first you may tire rapidly. Try to walk or do range-of-motion exercises each day for five minutes. As you comfortably can, add exercise or increase your pace. Add time gradually, until you exercise a minimum of 30 minutes at least five days each week. Keep your goals manageable. Perhaps you can only walk a minute each day at first. But if you add a minute each week, you'll be walking nearly an hour each day after a year. Slow down and let your muscles and heart rate return to normal during the final five to 10 minutes of each session.

Warning signs

It's important to listen to your body carefully when you have arthritis. You'll learn by trial and error how much is too much. Pay attention to how you feel before and after you exercise. Rule No. 1: If you feel the same or better, it's working. If you feel worse, it's not.

Introduce new activities gradually and heed warning signs. Seek emergency medical attention immediately if you experience chest pain, severe shortness of breath, faintness, dizziness or nausea. If

---

Gather your equipment

The most important equipment is a comfortable, supportive pair of athletic shoes appropriate for the exercise you do. Always replace shoes before wear causes foot pain. You can buy special handles for sports equipment — golf clubs and table tennis paddles, for example — and garden tools. An occupational therapist can advise you.

Be cautious about adding weights to your strength training program. Weights can aggravate joint pain and increase swelling, especially when your arthritis is very active. If you do use weight-training equipment, you don't have to spend a lot of money. Some athletic stores sell weights by the pound. Or check your newspaper's classified ads for used sets. Doctors and therapists often recommend that people with rheumatoid arthritis use light weights or exercise without weights.

---

exercise brings on a cramp or muscle pain, gently rub and stretch the muscle until the pain subsides. If the pain persists and your limb loses its color, see a doctor immediately.

Finish your session with slow, easy movements. If you experience new pain later in the day or fatigue the following day, you've probably done too much too fast or an inappropriate activity. You may need a new activity. Your doctor or physical therapist can advise you.

Recommended exercises

If you can walk, walking is your best bet for a starter exercise. If you can't walk, try a stationary bicycle with no resistance or do hand or arm exercises. It's good to move each joint in its full range of motion every day. The following descriptions may jog your memory of what you've learned in physical therapy. If you don't understand them, talk with your therapist or doctor or look for them on a recommended video.

Flexibility exercises

These exercises help maintain normal joint function and relieve stiffness. Do an assortment of them for five to 10 minutes several times each day. As you can, gradually add a few repetitions. Avoid pain.

Your neck:

- Bring your head forward, as though to touch your chin to your chest. Return your head upright. Use care with rheumatoid arthritis.
- Tilt your ear to your left shoulder without raising your shoulders. Return your head upright. Repeat to the right.
- Turn your face to the left, keeping neck, shoulders and trunk straight. Repeat to the right.

Your shoulders:

- With your arms at your side, roll your shoulders forward in a circular motion. Reverse.
- Stand with your feet shoulder-width apart. Hold a cane, broomstick or wand comfortably with both hands (1). Raise the cane forward and upward over your head (2). Return to the starting position. Repeat. You may place your palms up (as in illustration) or down.

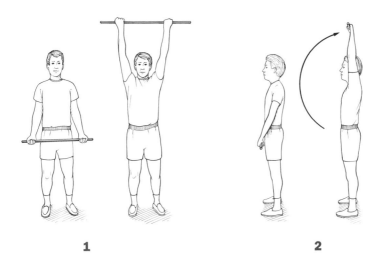

1 **2**

- To exercise one arm, hold the cane vertically in front of you. Place the arm to be exercised higher on the cane (3). Your lower arm may push to help raise your upper arm.

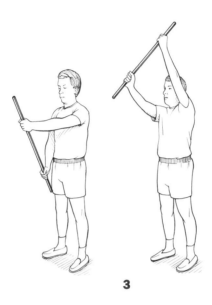

3

- Stand with your feet shoulder-width apart. Grasp the cane with both hands, palm up on the hand you are exercising (4). Raise your arm out to the side (not in front of you). Continue, until your arm touches your ear. Return to the starting position. Change hands and repeat (5).

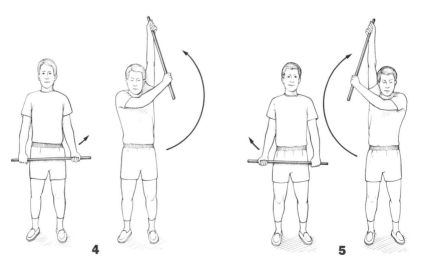

4   **5**

• Stand with your feet shoulder-width apart. Hold the cane behind your back, with your hands shoulder-width apart (6). Slowly move the cane backward and upward, keeping your elbows straight (7). All movement should come from your shoulders. Don't lean forward to get more motion. Return to the starting position. Repeat.

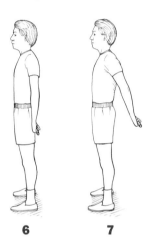

6   **7**

• With arms out to your sides, bend your elbows and hold the cane in front of your chest (8). Gently move the cane in an upward arc toward your head (9). Try not to move your upper arms. Repeat. Move the cane over your head and lower it to the base of your neck (10). Repeat.

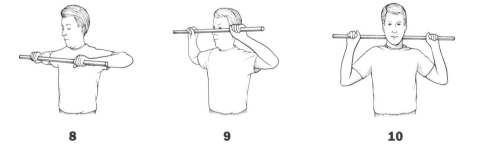

8   **9**   **10**

- With your arms out to your sides, bend your elbows and hold the cane in front of your chest (11). Gently move the cane in a downward arc toward your stomach (12). If you can, position the cane behind your hips, with your palms facing behind you. Slowly raise the cane up along your back toward your shoulder blades (13). Repeat.

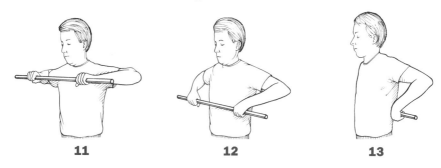

- With your upper arms against your body, bend your elbows and grasp the cane with palm up on the arm that will move outward (14). The palm on the arm that will move inward faces down. Gently slide the cane across your body so that one forearm swings outward from your body while the other one swings inward toward your stomach (15). Repeat. Change palm positions and repeat.

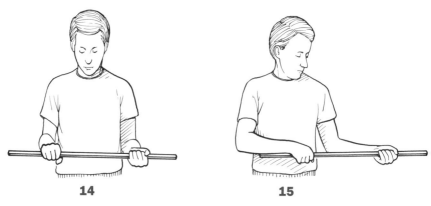

- Place your right palm behind your neck and the back of your left hand in the small of your back. Gently attempt to touch your hands behind your back. Reverse.

- Clasp your hands behind your head. Slowly breathe in as you gently move your elbows back and release your breath as you relax your elbows forward.
- Bring both elbows to shoulder height. Ease your elbows backward and feel a slight (not painful) stretch in your chest muscles.

Your hands and fingers:

- Bend your thumb across your palm to touch your little finger (16).
- Straighten your fingers (18). Relax and repeat with each hand. Make an "O" by touching your thumb to each fingertip (17). Open your hand wide (18). Relax and repeat.
- Bend and straighten the end and middle joints of your fingers (20). Keep your knuckles straight. Relax and repeat with each hand.
- Bend your fingers to make a fist. Bend each joint as much as possible (19). Relax and repeat with each hand.

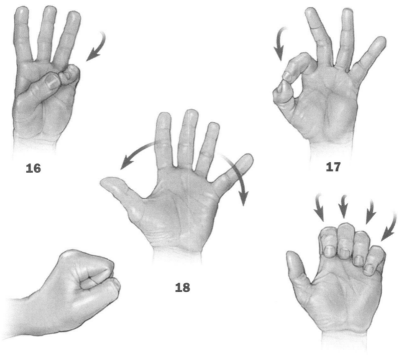

16

17

18

19

20

Your elbows:

• Bend both elbows, bringing your forearm up until your fingers touch your shoulders. Straighten arms.

• Keep your upper arms next to your body while bending your elbows to form a right angle. Turn your palms toward the ceiling, then toward the floor.

Your wrists:

• Keep your upper arms at your side and bend your elbows to form a right angle. Hold your hands out with your thumbs facing upward. Move both hands toward your stomach, then facing out as far as possible.

Your hips:

• While standing, lift your knee toward your chest to make a right angle. Alternate legs to march in place. Try this while lying on your back, too. Keep one leg extended as the other leg is bent. Grasp the back of the thigh of your bent leg and gently pull it toward your chest. Don't force your leg. Repeat with the other leg.

• Stand and face a chair. Hold onto the back of the chair for support. Gently move one straight leg out to the side and return. Repeat with the other leg. You can also do this exercise lying down, sliding one leg at a time out to the side and back to midline.

• Lie on your back, feet together, toes pointed up. Slide one leg to the side. Keep your toes pointed to the ceiling. Turn your foot in, then out. Return your leg to midline. Repeat with the other leg.

Your knees:

• Hold onto the back of a chair as you stand on one foot. Keep your knees together. Gently flex your knee and bring one foot up. Alternate. Don't arch your back. You can do this lying on your stomach, with a pillow supporting your stomach and hips. Keep one leg extended. Bring the other foot up toward

Remember:
Seek medical advice before you begin any exercise program. Your doctor or physical therapist can instruct you in exercises suited to your specific needs.

Your daily back routine

Walking is the most important way to exercise the muscles of your back. In addition to walking, a wide variety of exercises to stretch and strengthen your back and supporting muscles is available. A few of the most commonly prescribed maneuvers are shown here.

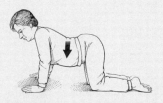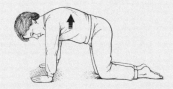

Cat stretch

Step 1: Get down on your hands and knees. Slowly let your back and abdomen sag toward the floor. Step 2: Slowly arch your back away from the floor. Repeat several times.

Half sit-up

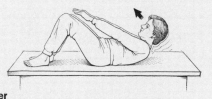

Lie on your back on a firm surface with your knees bent and feet flat. With your arms outstretched, reach toward your knees with your hands until your shoulder blades no longer touch the ground. Don't grasp your knees. Hold for a few seconds and slowly return to the starting position. Repeat several times.

Shoulder-blade squeeze

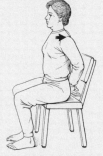

Sit upright on a chair. Keep your chin tucked in and your shoulders down. Pull your shoulder blades together and straighten your upper back. Hold a few seconds. Return to starting position. Repeat several times.

Leg lift

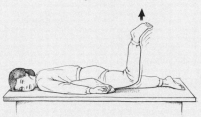

Lie face down on a firm surface with a large pillow under your hips and lower abdomen. Keeping your knee bent, raise one leg slightly off the surface and hold for about five seconds. Repeat several times.

the back of your thigh by bending your knee. Don't force your knee to an uncomfortable angle. Return your leg to an extended position. Repeat with the other leg.

* Lie on your back. Bend your knee to place one foot flat. Slide the heel as close to your buttock as possible, then extend. Repeat with the other leg.
* Sit in a chair with your ankles crossed. Push your feet against each other. Put the other foot in front and repeat.

Your calves:

* Stand an arm's length from the wall, with one foot forward. Place your hands on the wall at shoulder level (21). Keep your back straight as you lean toward the wall with your hips (but not to the point of pain). Relax and repeat with the other leg.

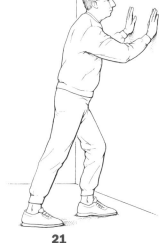

21

Your hamstrings:

* Sit in a chair with one leg on another chair (22). Keep your back straight. Slowly bend forward at your hip until you feel a slight stretch in the back of your thigh. Repeat with the other leg.

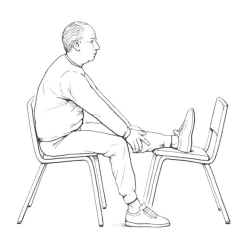

22

Your ankles and feet (skip these exercises if they are painful):
- Stand with your feet about 12 inches apart. Rise to your toes with both feet. Relax to the starting position. Rise to the toes of your right foot. Relax. Rise to the toes of both feet. Relax. Rise to the toes of your left foot. Relax. Repeat.
- Walk on your heels.
- Walk on your toes.
- Walk heel to toe, as if on a tightrope.
- While standing, lift your left foot and place it to the right of your right foot. Repeat with left foot planted, placing your right foot to the left of your left foot. This is called braiding.

Strength training

Studies have shown that strength training — also called resistance training — provides significant improvement in muscle strength, muscle endurance and contraction speed of muscles that support arthritic joints. Strength training also has been shown to provide pain relief for people with arthritis.

After warming up with flexibility exercises, try to do strength training several times a week, but only if you can do so without pain. Consider not using weights at first. As you gain strength, you may gradually add weight and repetitions. Isometric exercises, which involve no movement, can be very beneficial for people with arthritis.

- Chair sit-ups (23). Skip this exercise if your hands, wrists and elbows are painful. Sit in a sturdy chair that has arms (no wheels), with your feet firmly on the floor. Push your body up off the surface of the chair using your arms only. Relax and repeat.

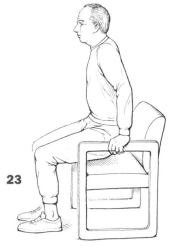

23

- Chair sits. Set up two chairs as shown (24). Lightly hold onto the chair in front of you. Begin to sit in the chair behind you in a position you can hold for five seconds. As you build strength, extend the hold time and try to hold a lower position that is almost, but not quite, seated. Relax and repeat. Don't plop down when you sit to rest.

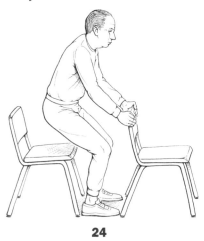

24

- Quadriceps. Sit or lie down on your back with one leg extended, foot supported and knee straight. Push your knee straight by tightening the muscles on the front of your thigh. Imagine that your leg is getting longer. Repeat with your other leg.
- Hamstring. Sit or lie down on your back with your knee slightly bent. Push down on your flat heel by tightening the muscles at the back of your thigh. Repeat with your other leg.
- Gluteus. Lie facedown, legs extended. Squeeze your buttocks together. Relax.
- Lie on your back, legs flat on the bed. Weave a belt snugly in a figure eight around both legs just above your knees (25). Pull with both legs equally to spread them apart as far as the belt allows, keeping toes, legs and knees extended straight. Relax.

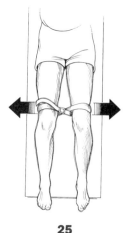

25

• Sit on the edge of a chair (26). Weave a belt snugly in a figure eight around both legs just above your knees. Pulling your legs in opposite directions, lift one leg up off the chair. Relax. Repeat with the other leg.

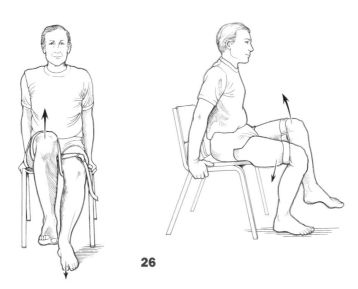

26

• Sit on the edge of a chair. Weave a belt snugly in a figure eight around both ankles (27). Attempt to straighten one knee while pulling the other foot backward, applying equal force with both legs. Relax. Repeat with the other leg.

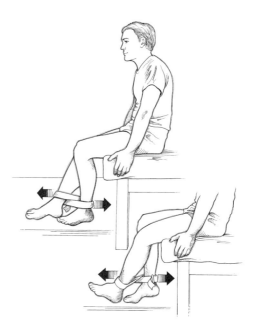

27

- Stand facing a wall, arms at your side (28). Keeping a straight elbow, move one arm forward and press the back of your hand against the wall. Repeat with the other hand.
- Stand sideways next to a wall, arms at your side (29). Push the back of the hand near the wall out to the side against the wall. Turn and repeat with your other hand.
- Stand with your back against a wall, arms hanging straight at your side (30). Keeping your elbow straight, push first one then the other arm back against the wall.

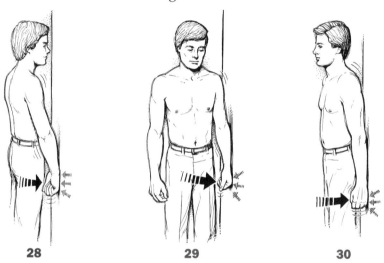

28   29   30

Aerobic training

Begin an aerobic exercise program gradually, slowly increasing the intensity and length of your workouts. Try to build up to at least 30 minutes of aerobic activity five or more days a week, adding a minute or two over a period of days or weeks. If you're comfortable with your level of activity and want an additional challenge, gradually increase to 45 to 60 minutes, five days a week. This approach promotes aerobic conditioning and appropriate body composition and helps prevent osteoporosis.

Use your exercise journal to periodically check your fitness level. Listen to your body. Use the resources available to you. A good exercise program not only can renew your energy but also may provide new fun and friends.

Chapter 12

Good nutrition and arthritis

The food choices you make each day can have a significant effect on your overall health and well-being, especially if you have arthritis. If you aren't eating a balanced diet, you may feel fatigued. Eating too much of the wrong kinds of foods can cause you to gain weight, which can worsen arthritis-related pain and lower your self-esteem. To feel healthy, it's important to eat healthy. A balanced diet can give you added energy and help you control your weight.

If you think of healthy eating as simply counting calories or tallying grams of fat, it's time to think about food in a new way. Eating well means enjoying great taste as well as healthy nutrition. No single food provides all of the nutrients your body needs. Eating a variety of foods helps ensure the right mix of nutrients for good health.

The basics

Experts agree that the best way to increase nutrients in your diet and limit fat and calories is to eat more plant-based foods. Plant foods — fruits, vegetables and foods made from whole grains — contain beneficial vitamins, minerals, fibers and health-enhancing

Body mass index (BMI)

BMI	Healthy		Overweight					Obese				
	19	24	25	26	27	28	29	30	35	40	45	50
Height						Weight in pounds						
4'10"	91	115	119	124	129	134	138	143	167	191	215	239
4'11"	94	119	124	128	133	138	143	148	173	198	222	247
5'0"	97	123	128	133	138	143	148	153	179	204	230	255
5'1"	100	127	132	137	143	148	153	158	185	211	238	264
5'2"	104	131	136	142	147	153	158	164	191	218	246	273
5'3"	107	135	141	146	152	158	163	169	197	225	254	282
5'4"	110	140	145	151	157	163	169	174	204	232	262	291
5'5"	114	144	150	156	162	168	174	180	210	240	270	300
5'6"	118	148	155	161	167	173	179	186	216	247	278	309
5'7"	121	153	159	166	172	178	185	191	223	255	287	319
5'8"	125	158	164	171	177	184	190	197	230	262	295	328
5'9"	128	162	169	176	182	189	196	203	236	270	304	338
5'10"	132	167	174	181	188	195	202	209	243	278	313	348
5'11"	136	172	179	186	193	200	208	215	250	286	322	358
6'0"	140	177	184	191	199	206	213	221	258	294	331	368
6'1"	144	182	189	197	204	212	219	227	265	302	340	378
6'2"	148	186	194	202	210	218	225	233	272	311	350	389
6'3"	152	192	200	208	216	224	232	240	279	319	359	399
6'4"	156	197	205	213	221	230	238	246	287	328	369	410

Note: Asians with a BMI of 23 or higher may have an increased risk of health problems.

Source: National Institutes of Health, 1998

FORMULA

You can calculate your exact BMI by using this formula:

$$\left(\frac{\text{Weight in pounds}}{(\text{ Height in inches }) \times (\text{ Height in inches })} \right) \times 703 = BMI$$

EXAMPLE

For example, if you weigh 165 pounds and you're 5 feet 10 inches tall, your BMI is 23.7.

$$\left(\frac{165 \text{ pounds}}{(70 \text{ inches }) \times (70 \text{ inches })} \right) \times 703 = 23.7$$

compounds called phytochemicals. Phytochemicals may help reduce the risk of chronic diseases, such as cardiovascular disease, diabetes and cancer. By emphasizing plant foods in your diet, you increase consumption of many naturally healthy compounds. Plant foods also are relatively low in calories — an added benefit for controlling weight.

A sensible approach to healthy weight

An effective diet to control weight may require you to reduce the number of calories you consume, but it shouldn't be at the cost of good health, taste and practicality. The diet you choose should be simple and inexpensive to follow. Otherwise, you won't stay with the plan. A diet that's enjoyable and satisfying is vital to the long-term success of your healthy weight program.

The Mayo Clinic Healthy Weight Pyramid is a guide to achieving a healthy weight while maintaining good nutrition. The pyramid is based on the concept of energy density. It promotes a plant-based diet, represented by the organization of the pyramid. The vegetables and fruits groups share the base of the pyramid — meaning you eat more of them than the other food groups — and the carbohydrates group is located just above them.

The Mayo Clinic Healthy Weight Pyramid can help you improve your health and achieve your weight goals. It's an easy-to-use guide to what you need to eat daily from each of six food groups, and it's geared to losing weight as well as maintaining weight.

A look at the food groups

The Mayo Clinic Healthy Weight Pyramid divides foods into six groups — vegetables, fruits, carbohydrates, protein and dairy, fats, and sweets. One of the first things you'll probably notice is that some of the groups carry the name of a type of food, such as vegetables, while others have the same name as a type of nutrient, such as carbohydrates.

In fact, most foods are a mixture of nutrients and don't fit neatly into categories. For the purposes of the pyramid, think of the

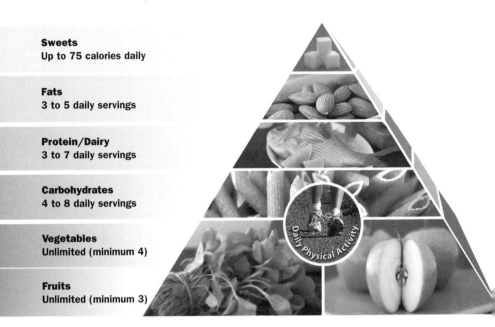

Sweets
Up to 75 calories daily

Fats
3 to 5 daily servings

Protein/Dairy
3 to 7 daily servings

Carbohydrates
4 to 8 daily servings

Vegetables
Unlimited (minimum 4)

Fruits
Unlimited (minimum 3)

Daily Physical Activity

Mayo Clinic Healthy Weight Pyramid

The Mayo Clinic Healthy Weight Pyramid is your guide to achieving and maintaining a healthy weight. It's triangular shape shows you where to focus your attention when selecting healthy foods. Eat more from the food groups at the bottom of the pyramid and less from those at the top.

See your doctor before you begin any healthy weight plan.

pyramid's building blocks as food groups rather than as particular nutrient types. These food groups point you in the right direction for eating a healthy, balanced diet.

The food groups of the Mayo Clinic Healthy Weight Pyramid are based on several factors. For one thing, the groups differ in their levels of energy density — the number of calories in a given quantity of a food. Foods that have few calories in a relatively large quantity of the food have a low energy density and form the base of the pyramid, meaning they form a larger part of your diet. Foods that have a high energy density (lots of calories for a given quantity) are a smaller block in the pyramid, meaning you eat less of them.

Foods within each group also share common health benefits to your overall diet, with foods at the base of the pyramid rich in variety and nutrients. The group breakdown is also practical in terms of your ability to select and prepare different foods.

Vegetables and fruits

Vegetables and fruits share many attributes. In fact, some foods that we term vegetable — such as tomatoes and cucumbers — are technically fruits. Both offer a wide array of flavors, textures and colors. They not only provide sensory pleasure but also many disease-fighting nutrients. Most vegetables and fruits are low in energy density because they are high in water and fiber, which provide no calories. You can improve your diet without reducing the amount of food you eat by eating more vegetables and fruits in place of foods that have more calories.

Vegetables. Vegetables include roots such as carrots and beets, tubers such as potatoes, members of the cabbage family, and salad greens such as lettuce and spinach. Other plant foods, such as peppers and eggplant (and others mentioned above), are included in this group, although technically they're fruits.

One serving of vegetables contains about 25 calories. In general, vegetables have less sugar (and therefore have fewer calories) and are less sweet tasting than fruits are. Vegetables contain no cholesterol, are low in fat and sodium, are high in dietary fiber and in essential minerals such as potassium and magnesium, and contain beneficial plant chemicals known as phytochemicals.

Fresh vegetables are best, but frozen vegetables are good, too. Most canned vegetables are high in sodium because sodium is used as a preservative in the canning process. If you use canned vegetables, look for labels that indicate that no salt is added, or be sure to rinse them.

Fruits. Any food that contains seeds surrounded by an edible layer is generally considered a fruit. In North America, fruits such as apples, oranges, peaches and plums, and slightly more exotic fruits such as mangos and papayas, are commonly available. These foods taste sweet or sweet-tart and are often eaten for snacks or desserts.

Like vegetables, fruits are great sources of fiber, vitamins, minerals and other phytochemicals. One serving equals about 60 calories and is virtually fat-free, so fruits can help you control your weight and reduce your risk of weight-related diseases. Fresh fruit is best, but frozen fruits with no added sugar and fruits canned in water or

Setting the record straight

Carbohydrates don't make you fat — excess calories do. Recently, many diets have promoted low-carbohydrate foods for weight loss. These diets claim that carbohydrates stimulate insulin secretion, which promotes body fat. So, the logic goes, reducing carbohydrates will reduce body fat. As a matter of fact, carbohydrates do stimulate insulin secretion immediately after they're consumed, but this is a normal process that allows carbohydrate building blocks such as glucose to be absorbed into cells. People who gain weight on high-carbohydrate diets do so because they're eating excess calories. Excess calories from any source, whether it contains a lot of carbohydrates or only a few, will cause weight gain.

Furthermore, some low-carbohydrate diets restrict grains, fruits and vegetables and emphasize the consumption of protein and dairy products, which can be high calorie and loaded with saturated fat and cholesterol. Plant-based foods not only are low in saturated fat and cholesterol-free but also are loaded with vitamins, minerals and other nutrients. These nutrients play a protective role in fighting serious diseases such as cancer, osteoporosis, high blood pressure and heart disease.

So be skeptical of the low-carbohydrate claims. Many carbohydrate-containing foods are healthy and can be an important part of a weight-loss plan.

their own juice are also excellent. Use fruit juice and dried fruits, such as raisins and prunes, sparingly because they're a concentrated source of calories. That is, they have a higher energy density.

Carbohydrates

Carbohydrates include an extensive range of foods that are a major source of energy for your body. Most carbohydrates are plant-based. These include grain products such as cereal, bread, rice and pasta. Carbohydrates may also come from other food groups, including starchy vegetables such as potatoes, corn, sweet potatoes and winter squash.

Carbohydrates provide a variety of nutrients and are generally low in fat and calories. One serving equals approximately 70 calories. Carbohydrates vary in energy density, depending on whether they're simple or complex substances. The more complex carbohydrates — for example, grains and grain products — have a moderately low energy density. They're often high in fiber. Be aware that foods such as croissants and dessert breads predominantly made from grain products also include other ingredients, such as fats, making them high in calories, therefore high in energy density.

When choosing grain products, look for the word *whole*, as in whole wheat, on the packaging and in the ingredients list. Whole grains contain the bran and germ, which are sources of fiber, vitamins and minerals. When grains are refined, some of the nutrients and the fiber are eliminated. As a rule, the less refined a carbohydrate, the better it is for you.

Protein and dairy

Proteins are essential to human life — every cell in your body contains them. Your skin, bone, muscle and internal organs are made up of proteins, and they're found in blood, hormones and enzymes. Proteins are important components of many foods. One serving of protein equals approximately 110 calories.

Foods rich in proteins and relatively low in fat and saturated fat include legumes, fish and lean meat. Legumes are a class of vegetables that include beans, peas and lentils. Legumes are typically low in fat, contain no cholesterol, and are high in protein, folate, potassium, iron and magnesium. Whole-milk dairy products are good sources of proteins and calcium but are high in fat, especially saturated fat. Low-fat or skim milk, yogurt and cheese have the same nutritional values as the whole-milk varieties but without the fat and its calories. They're relatively low in energy density, too, because they contain a lot of water.

Fats

Many people are surprised to hear that certain fats are essential to the life and function of the body's cells. Along with providing reserves of stored energy, these fats play a role in the immune system, help maintain cell structure, and play a role in the regulation of many body processes. In short, you need some fat in your diet.

Fats (lipids) are substances that don't dissolve in water. The fats group of the Mayo Clinic Healthy Weight Pyramid includes added fats, such as oils, margarine, butter, salad dressings and mayonnaise, and high-fat foods, such as avocados, olives, seeds and nuts. The fats group of the Pyramid doesn't include fat you get from eating animal products — meats, dairy products and eggs — which are the main sources of fat in the American diet.

There are several different kinds of fat in the food you eat, including saturated, polyunsaturated, monounsaturated and trans fats. In terms of healthfulness, not all fats are equal. The best fats are the monounsaturated varieties, such as olive oil and canola oil. But all fats contain approximately 45 calories a serving and are a high-energy-density food. For that reason, all fats, including the healthier ones, should be consumed sparingly.

Saturated fat. Saturated fat is the main dietary culprit in raising blood cholesterol and increasing the risk of disease in your body's coronary arteries. Foods high in saturated fat include red meats and most dairy products, as well as butter, lard, and coconut, palm and other tropical oils. Limit these fats and choose low-fat dairy products.

Polyunsaturated fat. This type of fat helps lower your blood cholesterol but is susceptible to a harmful process called oxidation. Safflower, corn, sunflower and soy oils are high in polyunsaturated fat. Cold-water fish, such as salmon, provide a heart-healthy form of this fat — omega-3 fatty acids. As noted in a later section, some studies suggest omega-3 fatty acids help control rheumatoid arthritis.

Monounsaturated fat. Monounsaturated fat helps reduce low-density lipoprotein (LDL) cholesterol and is more resistant to oxidation than the polyunsaturated fats. It also helps clear arteries by maintaining high-density lipoprotein (HDL) cholesterol. Nuts, avocados, canola oil, olive oil and peanut oil are sources of monounsaturated fat. These are the healthier fats to consume in your diet.

Trans fat. Also referred to as partially hydrogenated vegetable oil, this type of fat may be even more harmful to your health than

Average serving sizes

Below are the average serving sizes for food groups in the Mayo Clinic Healthy Weight Pyramid.

Food group	Average serving size	Calories per serving
Vegetables	2 cups leafy or 1 cup solid	25
Fruits	½ cup sliced or one medium piece	60
Carbohydrates	½ cup grain or 1 slice of bread	70
Protein and dairy	½ cup beans, 3 oz fish, 1 cup 2 percent milk, 1½ oz lean meat or 2 oz low-fat cheddar cheese	110
Fats	1 tsp oil or 2 tbsp nuts	45

saturated fat. Trans fat raises "bad" LDL cholesterol levels and lowers "good" HDL cholesterol, along with other effects. The most common sources of trans fat include margarine or shortening, and any products made from them, such as cookies, crackers and deep-fried foods.

Sweets

Foods in the sweets group of the Mayo Clinic Healthy Weight Pyramid include candies, cakes, cookies, pies, doughnuts and other desserts. And don't forget the table sugar you add to cereal, fruit, and beverages. Sweets are a high source of calories, mostly from sugar and fat, and are high in energy density, yet they offer little in terms of good nutrition. You don't have to give up these foods, but be smart about your selections and portion sizes. The pyramid recommends limiting sweets to 75 calories a day. Where possible, select better dessert choices, such as fig bar cookies and low-fat frozen yogurt.

Determining your servings for a healthy weight

The Mayo Clinic Healthy Weight Pyramid provides a range of servings for each food group. The number of servings you should eat within each range depends on a variety of factors, including your weight, activity level, age and whether you want to lose weight. If you're trying to lose weight, you'll want to aim for the lower number of servings in the food groups rather than the higher number. It's important, however, that you eat at least the minimum servings for each food group to maintain good health. A dietitian can help you determine how many servings of each food you should eat to maintain a calorie level that will help you lose weight.

As you adopt a healthier diet, it's also important to understand what constitutes a serving (see "Average serving sizes" on page 273). With the trend toward supersizing, all-you-can-eat buffets and huge portions in restaurants, many people have an inaccurate idea of what a serving is. Pay close attention to portion sizes so you know how many servings are in the portions you're eating. Don't just estimate. Practice at home by actually measuring cupfuls and spoonfuls and weighing some foods.

Menu planning

Many people say they don't plan menus, but everyone plans, if only for what to pick up at the grocery store. Planning menus means thinking about what foods to eat for a meal, a day or a week. There are many advantages to planning meals, and you don't have to lock yourself into a rigid schedule. Planning has these advantages:

- **Increases variety.** You can include new foods and vary the colors, textures, flavors and shapes of foods to make meals attractive and interesting. Planning can make it easier to choose foods that are low in fat and calories and high in nutrients.
- **Saves energy and money.** When you go to the grocery store, take advantage of precut fruits and vegetables, meats cut for stir-frys and other items that can save you time in the kitchen.

  They may cost a little more, but they're worth it when your energy is low or you're in pain. Even prepared foods from the grocery store are less expensive than take-out or restaurant foods of similar nutritional value.

Adding nutrition to convenience foods

Here are some easy nutritional fixes for convenience foods:

- Add fresh peppers, grated carrots, mushrooms and onions to canned spaghetti sauce to boost fiber and nutrients.
- Top frozen pizza with fresh tomatoes and your favorite vegetables before heating.
- When preparing packaged rice, toss in vegetables (peas, broccoli, corn) or fruit (raisins, apple, apricots).
- Serve fresh fruits and vegetables as extra side dishes when eating frozen microwave dinners.
- Add a bag of ready-to-eat leafy salad greens and a loaf of crusty whole-grain bread the next time you opt for deli foods.

Cooking with ease

When you have arthritis, the time you have to prepare a meal and the amount of preparation you're able to manage can be major factors in deciding what foods to serve.

Make use of energy-saving storage devices such as Lazy Susans and pegboards and buy easy-open containers to keep food and equipment handy. A small cart on wheels can save a lot of steps and energy. Use it to set and clear the table. Arrange one complete place setting at a time and work your way around the table. Use the cart to carry items back to the sink, or have family members carry, scrape and stack their own dishes. A dishwasher also can make clean up easier, if you have one.

If you immediately rinse all cooking utensils and equipment after use, you won't have as much scrubbing to do later. A small electric food processor is easy to clean and can allow you to effortlessly chop and dice foods and grate cheese.

When cooking, try these work-simplification techniques:

- Study and improve placement of utensils to save steps and motions.
- Gather utensils and necessary items from storage areas and the refrigerator using a cart.

- Slide heavy objects along the counter rather than lift them.
- Serve hot items from the stove rather than lift heavy pots and pans.
- Cook and serve in the same dish whenever possible.
- Use a slotted spoon to remove vegetables from water.
- Place a nonslip pad or wet cloth under a mixing bowl to help hold it stationary without gripping.
- Work on paper towels when preparing vegetables and fruits to ease the cleanup.
- Keep knives sharpened.
- Plan to have leftovers to freeze and heat at another time or that can be quickly served in a new way. For example, a roast can be used later in the week for a stir-fry meal or added to salad greens for lunch. Make a double batch of a casserole. Keep one in the freezer for a day when you're too tired to cook.

Eating out

When you eat out, don't let large portions, unfamiliar menus and tempting desserts discourage you from your commitment to healthy eating.

Here are key points to keep in mind:

- **Look carefully for your restaurant.** Eating out might be a special time when you can get meals that you're finding difficult to prepare. It's also an opportunity to eat well. Find a restaurant that offers a variety of foods, where it's more likely you can choose a low-fat, healthy meal that's high on taste. Establishments that prepare the food you order from start to finish are more likely to accommodate special requests. A telephone call ahead of time (during nonpeak restaurant hours) can help you choose a restaurant best suited to your needs.
- **Keep hunger under control.** Don't skip a meal on a day you're eating out. In fact, you may want to have a light snack of vegetables or fruit an hour or so before the meal to avoid overeating.

Restaurant portion control

How many calories and how much fat do you avoid when you cut the portion sizes of these restaurant foods by half?

Food	Original portion	Original calories and fat (grams)	Calories and fat (grams) saved by eating ½ portion
Butter	1 tbsp	102/11.5	51/5.75
Salad dressing (regular)	1 ladle (4 tbsp)	About 240/ about 24 (depending on type)	About 120/ about 12 (depending on type)
Tartar sauce	4 tbsp	160/14	80/7
Roasted chicken breast (with skin)	7 oz	386/15.2	193/7.6
Sirloin steak	12 oz	1,120/88	560/44
Prime rib	12 oz	1,440/124	720/62
Fish fillet (breaded and batter fried)	8 oz	528/28	264/14

- **Survey the selections.** Many restaurants have special listings for healthy eating. However, foods in the diet or light section still may have far more calories and fat than you might expect. Look for meals that contain little or no fat, small amounts of meat, poultry or fish, and lots of vegetables and low-fat carbohydrates, such as baked potato, brown rice or whole-grain bread.
- **Order wisely.** Ordering a la carte can be more expensive, but it lets you get just what you want. It has the advantage of variety and reduced quantity. Try making a meal out of broth-based (not creamed) soup or a salad and one appetizer. Look for appetizers that are broiled, baked or steamed, not fried. In addition, consider sharing a meal, or ask for a take-home box

to come with your food, so you can immediately remove half to take home for another time.

- **Speak up.** Ask your server to clarify unfamiliar terms or to explain how a dish is prepared. Request smaller portions and substitutions, such as fresh fruit for french fries, dressings and sauces on the side and dry broiling (not basted with oil or fat) instead of frying.
- **Cut out the condiments.** Taste your food before instinctively adding salt, butter, sauces and dressing. Well-prepared food often needs only minimal enhancement. Ask for sauces or dressing on the side. Then use the fork-dip-food technique. Dab your fork in the sauce and then pick up your food. This allows you to enjoy the sauce but limits the amount.

Special nutrition issues

Do foods such as red meat, citrus fruits, tomatoes (and other night-shade foods containing glycoalkaloids), aspartame and alfalfa sprouts aggravate rheumatic conditions? Questions such as this are frequently asked by people with arthritis. Because the symptoms of arthritis vary from day to day, it seems natural to think that what you eat might affect how you feel.

For a small number of people with arthritis, it's possible that sensitivities to certain foods may trigger or worsen symptoms. But no scientific evidence has consistently shown that any particular food or food group makes arthritis pain or inflammation any better or worse. The one exception to this is gout. (See "Gout and diet" on page 279.)

If you believe that a particular food increases your symptoms, it's probably OK to drop it from your diet. However, don't omit whole food groups or a large number of foods without first consulting a registered dietitian or your doctor. Without proper guidance, you could become deficient in nutrients that are important to maintaining your health. This, in turn, could affect your arthritis symptoms. Be skeptical of any diet that eliminates an entire group of foods or stresses only a few foods while eliminating others.

Gout and diet

Gout, a form of arthritis characterized by sudden, severe attacks of pain, redness and tenderness in your joints, is caused by an excessive level of uric acid in your blood (hyperuricemia). Uric acid is a waste product formed from the breakdown of purines. These are substances found naturally in your body as well as in certain foods.

Although medications have decreased the need for severe dietary restrictions in people with gout, some dietary changes can help lessen the severity of gout attacks. They may also be useful for people who have problems with gout medications.

To help relieve symptoms of gout, try these dietary tips:

- Limit the animal protein in your diet to no more than 6 ounces of lean meat, poultry or fish a day. High-protein foods increase the blood level of uric acid. Organ meats (liver, brains, kidney and sweetbreads), anchovies, herring and mackerel are particularly high in purines.
- Limit or avoid alcohol. Drinking too much alcohol interferes with the removal of uric acid from your body.
- Drink plenty of liquids — just not alcohol. Fluids can help remove uric acid from your body.
- Lose weight if you're overweight. Gradual weight loss will lessen the load on affected weight-bearing joints and may also decrease uric acid levels. But avoid fasting or rapid-weight-loss diets. They can increase uric acid levels in your blood. Also avoid low-carbohydrate diets that are high in protein and fat, which can increase the risk of hyper-uricemia and exacerbate gout.

Supplements and alternative diets

If you have arthritis, you may wonder about the helpfulness of particular supplements or diets touted to improve your symptoms.

The naturally occurring oils in some cold-water fish that are high in omega-3 fatty acids have gained popularity as an alternative treatment for rheumatoid arthritis. Research seems to support a general consensus that cold-water-fish oils can indeed reduce the pain, inflammation and joint tenderness caused by rheumatoid arthritis. Omega-3 fatty acids seem to somehow modify the inflammatory process.

You can build cold-water-fish oils into your diet by eating cold-water fish such as salmon, mackerel, herring or trout at least once a week. Or you can take fish oil supplements. In fact, some research suggests that after three to four months of taking both fish oil supplements and nonsteroidal anti-inflammatory drugs (NSAIDs), some people with rheumatoid arthritis may be able to reduce their NSAID dose. It's important, of course, to check with your doctor before taking any supplement or changing your medications.

Researchers have studied other sources of omega-3 fatty acids, such as leafy green vegetables, flaxseed oil and canola oil. But so far, there's no evidence that these foods provide any special benefit for people with rheumatoid arthritis. The omega-3 fatty acid in these foods, alpha linolenic acid, seems to have a different physiologic effect than the omega-3s found in fish oils. There's some evidence that other plant oils, such as borage oil and evening primrose oil, possibly may ease symptoms of rheumatoid arthritis. But most studies of these oils have been small and of short duration. More research is needed.

Scientists also are studying whether certain diets can reduce the severity of rheumatoid arthritis. Some research suggests that following a vegetarian diet might be a useful part of treating the disease. In one small Swedish study, people with rheumatoid arthritis who followed a strict vegetarian (vegan), gluten-free diet for at least nine months experienced a 10-fold reduction in symptoms, when compared with those who followed a balanced, nonvegan diet. In another small study, the benefits of a very low-fat, vegan diet were seen after only four weeks.

Other research suggests that reducing meat intake, but not eliminating it entirely, also may be beneficial. In one small study, people who followed a mostly vegetarian (two small servings of meat per week) diet for eight months had fewer tender and swollen joints than those eating a typical Western diet. When the researchers added fish oil supplements to the diet, the beneficial effects were

10 ways to spot junk claims about nutrition

Members of the Food and Nutrition Science Alliance (FANSA) offer these tips to help you evaluate information about healthy eating. Any of the following signs should raise a warning flag:

1. Recommendations that promise a quick fix
2. Dire warnings of danger from a single product or regimen
3. Claims that sound too good to be true
4. Simplistic conclusions drawn from a complex study
5. Recommendations based on a single study
6. Dramatic statements that are refuted by reputable scientific organizations
7. Lists of "good" and "bad" foods
8. Recommendations made to help sell a product
9. Recommendations based on studies that are published without first being reviewed by experts
10. Recommendations from studies that ignore differences among individuals or groups

even greater. In another small study, people with rheumatoid arthritis who followed a traditional Mediterranean diet for 12 weeks had less inflammation, improved physical function and improved vitality, compared with those following a typical Western diet. In general, the Mediterranean diet contains less red meat and more fish than the typical Western diet.

It's hard to know exactly why these diets may be effective in reducing symptoms of rheumatoid arthritis. Is it limiting or eliminating meat that makes the difference — or is it including more antioxidant-rich fruits and vegetables? Nevertheless, the results — though preliminary — are intriguing.

It's important to remember that most claims about supplements and special diets for arthritis have no basis in scientific fact. Before taking any supplement or drastically changing your regular diet, be sure to check with a registered dietitian or your doctor first. (See Chapter 7 for more information on complementary and alternative treatments.)

Benefits of a healthy weight

Research has shown that being overweight or obese increases your risk of osteoarthritis of the knee. Being overweight or obese also clearly makes the signs and symptoms of arthritis worse. Excess weight adds stress to your weight-bearing joints, especially your knees, aggravating pain, stiffness and inflammation. There's never a good time to be overweight, but when it comes to arthritis, the effects appear to be worse if you become overweight in early to mid-adulthood. In one Finnish study, for example, normal weight people who became consistently overweight between age 20 and age 50 were two to three times more likely to need knee surgery for arthritis than were people who maintained a normal weight throughout those years.

The good news is that if you have osteoarthritis or rheumatoid arthritis and you're carrying extra weight, shedding some of those excess pounds can reduce stress on your back, hips, knees and feet — all places where you may feel pain. A decrease of just 5 percent to 10 percent in weight may:

- Decrease pain
- Provide a sense of control
- Increase mobility
- Increase ability to exercise
- Increase energy level
- Improve balance, which may
- Decrease fatigue
- Prevent falls
- Improve self-image

One Danish study, for example, tracked obese older adults with osteoarthritis of the knee who lost 10 percent of their weight over an eight-week period. The result? Reduced knee pain and a 28 percent improvement in the physical function of their knees.

Weight loss is especially important if you and your doctor are considering joint surgery, because excess weight can make the procedure more difficult and risky. In fact, some surgeons insist that their overweight patients lose weight before they undergo elective operations.

Weight control basics

The adage "You are what you eat" is only partially true. Other factors play a role as well:

- **Food intake.** Your intake of calories and the number of calories your body needs for energy (calories burned) influence your weight. If calorie consumption from foods is greater than your energy needs, weight gain will occur over time.

- **Body composition.** Lean muscle mass is your fat-free body weight. Lean muscle mass is important because it burns more calories than does fat tissue, making weight control easier. Exercise is the only proven method of increasing lean muscle tissue.

- **Calories are burned through activity.** If the number of calories you consume is less than the amount of energy you use, the result will be weight loss. Try to keep active. Inactivity results in weight gain — if your food intake remains constant — which may in turn cause further pain. This can lead to more

Mix and match for better health

Spending about 40 minutes in any combination of these activities burns at least 90 calories. Try to be this active on most days.

Activity	Calories burned in 10 minutes of activity*
Strolling (less than 2 mph)	23
Light housework (polishing furniture)	28
Ballroom dancing	34 to 62 (depends on intensity)
Bowling	34
Walking at a brisk pace	43
Bike riding	45 to 91 (depends on intensity)
Golfing (carrying bag)	50
Swimming, slow crawl	91

*Calories are based on a 150-pound person. If you weigh less than 150 pounds, you need to spend more time to use up the same number of calories. Weighing more than 150 pounds means you use up the same number of calories in less time.

> **Being underweight a risk with rheumatoid arthritis**
>
> Being overweight can worsen symptoms of arthritis. But for people with rheumatoid arthritis, there may be a greater risk in being too thin — even a risk of death.
>
> In a study conducted at Mayo Clinic, researchers found that people with rheumatoid arthritis who had a low body mass index (BMI) at the time of their diagnosis were more than three times as likely to die of cardiovascular disease, when compared with normal weight individuals without rheumatoid arthritis. Those with rheumatoid arthritis who were normal weight when diagnosed but then lost weight had about double the risk of cardiovascular death.
>
> Mayo Clinic doctors say it's likely that people with the most severe forms of rheumatoid arthritis have very active, systemwide inflammation, which can be associated with weight loss. For these people, they say, the best course of action is to find a physician who will pay close attention to cardiovascular disease prevention and care.

inactivity and result in a cycle of weight gain that is difficult to break.

Eating well can help you control weight, but adding regular moderate physical activity is just as important. Even with arthritis, there are many activities to choose from that can help burn calories and increase muscle mass. Normal daily activities such as cleaning, shopping and doing laundry help burn calories, too. Strengthening exercises, such as weight training, counteract muscle loss due to aging. The more active you are, the easier it is to maintain and even increase your muscle mass and keep a healthy weight. (See Chapter 11 for more information on exercise.) On days when you're not feeling well, try to choose lower intensity activities.

Calcium and osteoporosis

If arthritis causes you to be inactive for extended periods of time, you may have an increased risk of developing osteoporosis, the "brittle bones" disease, because inactivity can lead to calcium loss from bone. You're also at increased risk of developing osteoporosis if you have a type of inflammatory arthritis or connective tissue disease, such as rheumatoid arthritis or lupus, or if you take corticosteroid medications.

Each year, more than 1.5 million Americans have fractures related to osteoporosis. Most fractures occur in the hip, spine or ribs, but the disease can affect any bone in your body.

Getting enough calcium in your diet may help slow bone loss and reduce your risk of osteoporosis. In addition, you also need vitamin D to enhance the amount of calcium that ultimately reaches your bones. Your body makes vitamin D when sunlight converts a chemical in your skin into a usable form of this nutrient. Supplements may be appropriate for people who don't get enough calcium and vitamin D in food, who live in cloudy environments or who rarely go outside.

The recommended intakes for calcium and vitamin D are listed below. Although it's best to meet your needs for these bone-saving

Recommended daily intake of calcium and vitamin D for men and women

Age (years)	Adequate intake of calcium (milligrams/day)	Upper limit (milligrams/day)	Adequate intake of vitamin D (international units/day)	Upper limit (international units/day)
19 to 50	1,000	2,500	200 (5 micrograms)	2,000
51 to 70	1,200	2,500	400-600 (10-15 micrograms)	2,000
71 and older	1,200	2,500	600-800 (15-20 micrograms)	2,000

There is consensus among many physicians that a goal of 1,500 mg of calcium a day is reasonable for postmenopausal women.

nutrients with a well-chosen diet, many people fail to do so. It's important to include at least two servings of high-calcium foods every day. If you frequently miss this mark, check with your doctor or registered dietitian about the need for supplemental calcium and vitamin D.

Regular weight-bearing exercise such as walking or strength training also helps keep bones strong. The greater the demands you place on bone, the stronger and denser it becomes.

Medications for osteoporosis

In addition to dietary measures, several medications are available to promote stronger bones. Hormone therapy, often referred to as HT, is the best-known way to prevent osteoporosis in women. But not all effects of HT are positive. Taking HT as a combination thera-

15 best sources of calcium

Along with three cups of milk, a serving or two of any of these foods will provide at least 1,000 milligrams (mg) of daily calcium.

Food	Calcium (mg)
Tofu set with calcium, 1/2 cup	434
Fruit yogurt, 1 cup (average of low-fat brands)	345
Rice (calcium-fortified), 1 cup	300
Milk (skim and low-fat), 1 cup	298
Orange juice (calcium-fortified), 1 cup	240
Mozzarella cheese (part-skim), 1 oz	222
Canned salmon with bones, 3 oz	203
Ready-to-eat cereal (calcium-fortified), 1 cup	200 to 1,000 (check label)
Ricotta cheese (part skim), 1/4 cup	167
Bread (calcium-fortified), 2 slices	160
Spinach, 1/2 cup cooked	145
Cottage cheese (1% fat), 1 cup	138
Navy beans, 1 cup cooked	126
Parmesan cheese, 2 tbsp	111
Turnip greens, 1/2 cup cooked	100

py — estrogen plus progestin — can result in serious side effects and health risks.

If HT isn't for you, other prescription drugs can help slow bone loss and may even increase bone density over time. Alendronate (Fosamax) and risedronate (Actonel) are bisphosphonates that inhibit bone loss. They're often used to prevent osteoporosis in people who require long-term steroid treatment for arthritis. In general, bisphosphonates may reduce your risk of hip and spine fractures by about 50 percent. Raloxifene (Evista) is a medication that mimics estrogen's beneficial effects on bone density in postmenopausal women, without some of the risks associated with estrogen. Calcitonin (Miacalcin) is a hormone that acts on bone, usually administered in the form of a nasal spray. It's generally used to treat people with osteoporosis who are at high risk of fracture but can't take bisphosphonates or raloxifene. Tamoxifen, a synthetic hormone used to treat and prevent breast cancer, has an estrogen-like effect on bone cells. As a result, it appears to reduce the risk of osteoporotic fractures, especially in women over age 50.

Food and drug interactions

Just as the foods you eat can alter the effectiveness of some medications, some medications can interfere with how well your body uses nutrients. You may need higher-than-usual amounts of certain vitamins or minerals, depending on the medications you're taking. Often you can choose foods that provide the extra nutrients you need. Sometimes, your doctor may recommend a supplement.

How and when to take your medication should be thoroughly understood. Some of the drugs used to treat arthritis are most effective if you take them on an empty stomach, but others should be taken with food to prevent stomach irritation. Carefully follow the instructions of your doctor and pharmacist.

Some of the most common side effects of arthritis medications include heartburn and an upset stomach, often described as a gnawing pain or empty feeling in the stomach. These symptoms can be caused by food, medication or a combination of both. Sit upright for at least 15 to 30 minutes after meals and taking medications. Try to avoid eating for at least one hour before bedtime. Limit foods that tend to trigger reactions, such as alcohol, caffeine, colas, spicy foods, fried foods and ground black and red cayenne pepper.

Appetite control

The long-term use of particular drugs may increase your appetite, making it more difficult to keep your weight under control. Eat slowly and stretch mealtimes to a minimum of 20 to 30 minutes to allow your natural appetite control mechanism to work. Increasing the amount of high-fiber foods can help you feel full sooner. To get more fiber, try whole-grain breads instead of white bread, fresh fruit instead of juice and raw vegetables in place of cooked vegetables.

Try these additional tips to help appease an overactive appetite:

- **Eat breakfast.** Eating regular meals and snacks prevents the "famine-then-feast" syndrome. Make breakfast a high-fiber cereal, whole-grain bread and fresh fruit, and you may feel less tempted to eat fatty, sugary snacks in the morning. It can also set you up for eating a more balanced lunch.
- **Be sure you're hungry.** Are you eating because you're stressed or bored? Substitute reading, a physical activity or a phone call to a friend.
- **Eat slowly.** Savor each flavor and texture to boost your satisfaction. Remember, it takes about 20 minutes for your brain to receive the signal that you're full. Make sure your meals last at least this long.
- **Ride out the urge.** Cravings generally pass within minutes, maybe even seconds. Busy yourself with an activity unrelated to food until the desire to eat passes.
- **Start small.** If you always finish what's in front of you, start with half the amount of food you usually eat on your plate. You may find smaller servings more satisfying. To make less food seem like more, serve your main course on a salad or dessert plate.
- **Enjoy a treat now and then.** If you're really committed to eating less, an occasional lapse is OK. It has little impact on a lifetime plan for controlling your appetite.

Chapter 13

Your thoughts, feelings, beliefs and your health

Because your mind and body are integrally connected, your beliefs about yourself, your arthritis and life itself have a powerful influence on you and your health. Whether you're optimistic or pessimistic, whether you think you have control and whether you have confidence in yourself affect how you approach life and how well you cope.

Put simply, positive or optimistic thoughts and beliefs can have health-enhancing benefits. Optimists are convinced they can make things work out. If you're an optimist, your positive attitude may buffer you from stress because you react to adversity by taking action. You face life's difficulties with a sense of hope. But negative or pessimistic thoughts and beliefs can intensify your stress and pain.

The mind-body connection works in many ways. First, if you believe you have control, you'll take better care of yourself — such as eating right, exercising and getting enough rest — than if you think nothing you do matters. Second, studies show that feelings of helplessness weaken the immune system by inhibiting the actions of T cells and natural killer cells, both of which attack invaders such as bacteria, viruses and tumor cells. Third, pessimistic people tend to isolate themselves, cutting themselves off from the proven health-enhancing benefits of friendship, love and support.

For arthritis in particular, research indicates that how you fare in managing your disease depends at least as much on your own actions as on those of your doctor and other health professionals. If you believe you can manage your arthritis — if you believe you can gain control over your pain and fatigue — then you're more likely to use medical resources more effectively than are people who have no faith in their ability to fight the disease. In fact, if you and some-one else have the same degree of physical impairment and you have developed better coping skills, you're likely to experience less pain and have less difficulty functioning.

It has taken years of research for science to prove what you learned as a child. If, like Chicken Little, you believe the sky will fall, you can subject your body to a constant state of damaging stress, increase your feelings of helplessness and make your day-to-day existence more difficult. But if, like the Little Engine That Could, you believe in yourself and your abilities, you can accomplish amazing things, such as managing your arthritis and living a full and satisfying life despite it. The choice is yours.

The healer within

Psychoneuroimmunology (si-koe-noor-o-imu-NOL-o-jee) is a field of study concerned with the interplay among stress, emotions, the nervous system, immune functions and disease. Your immune system's job is to maintain your health and facilitate healing by warding off invaders, such as viruses, and battling abnormal cells. Your nervous system plays its role in immune functioning by providing the communications link between your spleen, lymph nodes and thymus — organs that are part of the immune system — and through the release of hormones.

When you're stressed, your body gears up to either fight or flee by triggering areas of your brain to release hormones into your bloodstream. You know the feeling. When you're scared or excited, your heart beats faster, your breathing speeds up and your muscles tense. Those reactions can give you the boost you need to pass a test or give a speech. They can even "rev up" your immune system, preparing your body for injury or infection. But there's a downside. Research shows that when stress becomes long-term, or chronic, the chemicals your body releases can suppress your immune system, making you more susceptible to illness. If you're older or already have an illness, you're more prone to these stress-related changes.

When you have a chronic condition such as arthritis, stress can make it harder for you to deal with challenges. Perhaps one of the worst effects of stress is that the resulting muscle tension can worsen your pain by causing muscle fatigue. This, in turn, may reduce your stamina, cause you to feel helpless and intensify other feelings you might have, such as anger, anxiety, annoyance or frustration. As a result, you might become depressed, which makes you feel more helpless, setting up a painful cycle.

Stress is simply part of life, and you have no control over many stressful occurrences, such as the death of a loved one. Even positive events, such as a promotion or a wedding, can cause stress. For most of us, however, minor stressors are more common than major events. Research has shown that these minor events play a significant role in how you feel day to day. But stress also comes from within, and it's how you react to external situations that determines the level of stress you experience. Fortunately, you can learn to manage your stress.

Listening to your body

The first step in breaking the cycle — stress, increased pain, decreased abilities and depression — is learning to recognize when you're under stress. People experience stress differently. Some develop physical problems, while others experience emotional changes or changes in behavior.

Physical signs and symptoms of stress may include:
- Headache
- Chest pain
- Pounding heart
- High blood pressure
- Shortness of breath

- Muscle aches, such as back and neck pain
- Clenched jaws
- Grinding teeth
- Tight, dry throat
- Indigestion
- Constipation or diarrhea
- Stomach cramping or bloating
- Increased perspiration, often causing cold, sweaty hands
- Fatigue
- Insomnia
- Weight gain or loss
- Diminished sex drive
- Skin problems, such as hives

The mental or emotional effects of stress may include:

- Anxiety
- Restlessness
- Worrying
- Irritability
- Depression
- Sadness
- Anger
- Mood swings
- Feelings of insecurity
- Lack of concentration
- Confusion
- Forgetfulness
- Resentment
- A tendency to blame others for how you feel
- Guilt
- Pessimism

Stress can also cause changes in behavior. Signs and symptoms may include:

- Overeating or loss of appetite
- Decreased anger control, marked by sudden outbursts with little provocation
- Increased use of alcohol and drugs
- Increased smoking

- Withdrawal or isolation
- Crying spells
- Changes in close relationships
- Job dissatisfaction
- Decreased productivity
- Burnout

If you develop any of these problems, first try to determine whether they're not caused by something else. Once you determine, possibly with the help of your doctor or psychologist, that your symptoms are indeed stress-related, try to figure out what's causing them. Obviously, situations such as divorce or a death in the family are major stressors. But what about the day-to-day occurrences that rev up your stress reactors?

Take note of things that make your heart beat faster and boost your blood pressure. Is it arguing with a co-worker, sitting in rush-hour traffic, juggling too many commitments or maybe all of these? Try keeping a stress diary for a few weeks to get a better handle on what sets your nerves on edge.

Once you identify your symptoms and what triggers them, you can begin to control your stress, either by changing the situation, if possible, or by altering your reaction to it.

Focus on the positive

OK, so you have arthritis. That's no reason to think of yourself as unhealthy.

Remember, you have choices. Taking care of yourself, by eating the right foods, exercising and getting enough rest, will go a long way toward making you feel better and keeping you active. But what if you don't believe you have control over your situation? Chances are your automatic thoughts are working against you.

Rapid-fire or automatic thoughts pass through your brain constantly, although you may not be aware of most of them. If you stop and attend to your thoughts for a moment, you might be surprised how negative your self-talk can be. For example, you start a walking program and instead of focusing on the good you're doing yourself, you chide yourself for being out of shape. Or before you give a presentation at work, you tell yourself, "I can't," "I'm no good at this," or "They'll think I'm stupid." These are called automatic thoughts. Much stress comes from such negative thinking, which is usually unrealistic and distorted.

Psychologist Albert Ellis, the originator of rational-emotive therapy, said stress mostly develops not from what happens to us but from how we react to it. Our reactions are largely determined by irrational beliefs we hold, such as, "I should never make a mistake," "Everyone should like me," and "It's always wrong to get angry." Notice the "should," "always" and "never." Developing more realistic expectations for yourself and others through modifying these irrational beliefs is a powerful way to reduce stress.

You have to make yourself aware of your beliefs about yourself and understand how they trigger automatic thoughts. Begin to pay attention to what you're telling yourself. In regard to your arthritis, do you find yourself asking, "Why me?" and telling yourself that life as you knew it is over? When you catch yourself in the act of negative self-talk, stop, take a deep breath and think about the effect your thoughts are having on you. Use positive self-talk to tone down your critical or negative thinking. For example, instead of, "I'll never again be able to do the things I enjoy," tell yourself, "I'll take good care of myself so that I can still do many things" or "I may have to slow down, but I don't have to give up." By changing your view of a situation and your view of yourself, you may be able to find more constructive ways to cope.

David Burns, M.D., a psychiatrist and clinical associate professor at the Stanford University School of Medicine, believes that moods, including depression, result from the way you think about events, not the events themselves. He recommends restructuring negative thinking by writing down your negative thoughts as they occur. When you do something you consider a personal failure, such as needing help opening a jar, write down the thoughts that go through your head. Then counter them with a defense. For example, if your thought is, "I'm always such a burden on everyone," replace it with a more objective, rational one, such as, "Some days are better than others. Today I need more help." Tell the truth, because to change your reactions, you have to believe the rational thoughts. Dr. Burns suggests using this technique 15 minutes a day for several months to begin to replace automatic distortions with rational thinking.

9 tips for decreasing stress

In addition to redirecting stress-inducing thoughts, there are several other strategies for managing stress. You may talk about your problems with others, listen to some soothing music or sit in a warm bathtub or hot tub at the end of the day. Most of the time you may do pretty well in getting through life's crises as they arise. But at times you probably could do better.

The following tips may help you better manage stress:

- **Try to become more tolerant — of yourself and of situations over which you have no control.** Accepting that you'll always experience a certain degree of stress, and that this is normal, is helpful in managing stress.
- **Plan your day.** It may help you feel more in control of your life. Keep a schedule of your daily activities so that you're not faced with conflicts or last-minute rushes to get to an appointment or activity on time.
- **Get organized.** De-clutter your home and work space so that you don't have to spend time and energy looking for things you've misplaced.
- **Manage your time.** Often, stress is a result of too much to do and too little time. Setting priorities and practicing some simple time management skills may go a long way toward depressurizing your day.
- **Take occasional breaks.** Periodically during the day, take time to relax, stretch or walk.
- **Get adequate sleep, stay physically active and eat well.** A healthy body helps promote good mental health. Sleep helps you tackle problems with renewed vigor. Physical activity helps burn off stress-related tension. And a balanced diet provides you with energy to handle daily stress.

The unexpected benefits of treating depression

When you have arthritis, it's not unusual to also become depressed. If you're reluctant to seek treatment for depression, consider this: It could help improve your arthritis symptoms. A recent study, reported in the *Journal of the American Medical Association*, found that for older adults with both arthritis and depression, taking antidepressant medications or attending therapy sessions, or both, reduced their depressive symptoms and their arthritis pain. Study participants receiving treatment for depression also reported better joint function, overall health and quality of life.

- **Discuss your concerns.** Talking with a friend or family member may help to relieve stress and put events in perspective.
- **Get away.** Take a break from your normal routine and enjoy a change of scenery or a different pace.
- **Enjoy a good laugh.** It's healthy to spend time with people who have a positive outlook, take themselves lightly or have a sense of humor. Laughter helps reduce or relieve tension.

If self-help measures don't reduce your stress, help from a counselor, psychiatrist, psychologist or clergyperson may be what you need. Many people mistakenly believe that seeking outside help is a sign of weakness. But it takes strength to realize that you need help and good judgment to seek it.

Experimenting with relaxation techniques

Several specific techniques are designed to help you relax. As noted earlier, relaxing helps reduce the muscle tension that can increase pain. Finding a relaxation technique or techniques that work for you can help you decrease your pain and increase your comfort level.

Relaxation techniques need to be learned, which means practicing them regularly. Yoga and other techniques involving defined postures and repetitive movements can help you relax. Prayer and meditation, especially when kept simple, familiar and repetitive, may also help. These quiet, repetitive exercises can serve to reverse the mental arousal from stress. Regular practice also may provide new insights into how to reduce your stress by changing your priorities or thought patterns because these exercises serve as another powerful form of thought shifting.

What follows is a look at some of the more common relaxation techniques. There are many guided meditation and guided imagery products on the market that you may find helpful. Pick a quiet time and place where you won't be disturbed. Practice regularly, preferably daily, for a minimum of 15 to 20 minutes. And try to be patient — it may take several weeks to get the hang of it and start to see some benefit.

Meditation

This has been called an altered state of consciousness and a unique state of relaxation. There are almost as many ways to meditate as there are people who meditate. The basic premise is to sit quietly and focus on your breathing or on a simple word or phrase repeated over and over. When distracting thoughts arise — and they will — you simply notice them and let them go, always returning to your focus. With meditation, you enter a deeply restful state that reduces your body's stress response. Types of meditative practice include mindfulness meditation, the relaxation response and transcendental meditation. They work similarly. Regular practice of meditation can relax your breathing, slow brain waves and decrease muscle tension and heart rate. It can also lessen your body's response to the chemicals it produces when you're stressed, such as adrenaline, which can have harmful effects on your body.

Guided imagery (visualization)

This is a technique in which you enter a relaxed state brought on by meditation or self-hypnosis. There you imagine a setting you experience with your senses to help you alleviate physical symptoms. Studies of the brains of people engaged in guided imagery sessions suggest that the same parts of your brain are stimulated when you imagine something as when you actually experience it. The

A family matter

My three young sons and I all have rheumatoid arthritis. My wife, Nicki, is the only one in the family without the disease.

I've had arthritis since I was six weeks old. A swollen left elbow was the first clue. Thirty years later this was also the first clue for our oldest son, Timothy, when he was 3 months of age. He's now 8. Our twins, Jacob and Paul, developed the symptoms when they were 1. They're now 5.

Sometimes at our house, stress soars off the scale. It can happen in the morning when we're struggling to get one of the boys ready to go to the doctor to have swollen joints drained or injected with steroids. It can be hard to find the energy for patience when you've been up all night with them, soaking their flaring joints. But sometimes even those nights become divine, as we sit in the hot tub under the starlight and talk for hours about everything from knock-knock jokes to why Timothy can't play soccer anymore and how his courage inspires Mom and me.

We cope with the stresses. When there are a lot of swellings going on and things start to get crazy, we back away from activities.

message your brain receives from your imagination is sent to other brain centers and to your body's autonomic and endocrine systems, which regulate key functions such as heart rate and blood pressure.

Progressive muscle relaxation

This works on the theory that to learn how to relax your muscles, you must know how they feel tensed. Therefore, progressive relaxation is a series of exercises that takes you through each of the major muscle groups from head to toe — tensing and releasing tension as you go. Along the way, you focus on how the relaxed muscles feel compared with the tense muscles. Another important phase of progressive muscle relaxation involves a technique called body scanning, in which you focus on each muscle group in turn, note any tension and then let it go without first tensing the muscles.

Timothy hasn't been to Cub Scouts much this year, and he didn't make it to soccer, although we paid the $50 fee — just in case. We often, at the last minute, have to cancel holiday gatherings with family and friends. We've taken Timothy to counseling to help him over the depression he felt. Nicki and I also go to counseling to keep our marriage strong enough to endure the stresses created by the arthritis. Our friends have been a great help, too, watching the kids and running errands. Once, during an especially tough time, they brought meals for three months.

Nicki has a unique way of looking at our family's arthritis. She says the disease has shaped me into a "positive, focused, creative, wonderful person." And she tells our boys that it can do the same for them, if they decide to journey with arthritis instead of thinking of themselves as victims. For victims can only grow bitter, but travelers grow stronger each day.

Kevin
Arlington, Texas

Self-hypnosis

Self-hypnosis is an induced state of relaxation that enhances your focus and can help to make you more open to act on suggestions given to you — or that you give yourself — when you're in a hypnotic state. Self-hypnosis alters your brain wave patterns in much the same way as other relaxation techniques. This stress-relieving result may be why it works to ease pain and stress and alter behavior. About 75 percent of adults can be hypnotized.

Massage therapy

Massage therapy involves the manipulation of soft tissues of your body. There are several forms of massage therapy. They include the traditional kneading and rubbing of Swedish massage to the application of pressure at the acupuncture points of the body, which characterizes shiatsu massage. Massage can reduce your heart rate, increase circulation, relax muscles, improve range of motion and increase production of endorphins, which can relieve pain and anxiety. Massage is effective at relieving stress, depression and anxiety. It can also decrease pain perception. It has been shown to reduce arthritis pain. The environment in which you receive massage is important. A warm, quiet area, free from distracting noise or interruptions, can help relieve muscle tension. Low-volume sound or music also relaxes muscles. Your massage therapist may use a lubricant, such as mineral oil. By reducing friction, the lubricant contributes to smooth, effective massage strokes. Avoid a massage if you have an open wound or skin infection.

Keep a journal

Writing down your thoughts and feelings can help you blow off steam, increase self-awareness, solve problems and put things in perspective. The Arthritis Foundation recommends keeping a journal. By doing so regularly, you can also create a record of your symptoms, see patterns in their occurrence, gain a better understanding of your disease and find ways to communicate better with your doctors and others about your condition. You may also be able to determine whether your medications are affecting your mood or whether your arthritis flares when you're under stress. According to the Arthritis Foundation, people with chronic illnesses who record their feelings often report fewer symptoms, fewer doctor visits, fewer days off work and improved moods.

Seeking support — You're not alone

Having friends and loved ones to talk to, especially when you're facing the pain and changes arthritis impose on you, can help you feel less alone and scared and more able to cope with your condition. Having people who care about you also makes you more likely to take better care of yourself. In addition, studies show that having support may help improve your physical functioning and lower your level of psychological distress. Receiving daily friendliness and understanding from others may improve your psychological well-being. And having the social companionship of others — being asked to join in — appears to be beneficial both physically and psychologically.

Research also shows that support groups offer similar benefits, with one possible advantage: In a group of relative strangers, you can express your deepest fears and daily concerns without worrying about scaring or burdening your loved ones. Depending on the nature of the group, you can deal with difficult problems, get help changing your perspective, share ideas and experiences and learn more about arthritis and how others cope with the same challenges. To gain the most benefit from a group, it helps to be willing to share your thoughts and feelings and be interested in learning about those of others. To find a group, talk to your doctor, your local Arthritis Foundation chapter or others you know who have arthritis.

If you're not comfortable being in a group but feel the need to express your feelings about your arthritis or want help learning meditation or self-hypnosis, you might consider individual counseling. Talk to your doctor about recommended therapists.

Intimacy and arthritis

Sexuality is a natural and healthy part of living, and a part of your identity as a man or woman. But when the chronic pain of arthritis invades your life, the pleasures of sexuality often disappear. You may be concerned that sexual intercourse will cause you physical pain, especially if you have arthritis in your back or hip. You may be worried that your partner is less attracted to you because of your pain or swollen joints. Or you may have simply lost interest in sex as a result of pain, fatigue or other stresses associated with your condition.

Research suggests that two-thirds of people with osteoarthritis of the hip have sexual difficulties. Among those with rheumatoid arthritis, about half experience reduced sex drive and 60 percent are dissatisfied with their sex lives. But it doesn't have to be this way. You can have a healthy and satisfying sexual relationship, even when you have arthritis. The key is honest communication. It also helps to be creative and willing to make changes.

No matter what your health condition, it's important not to lose sight of your sexuality. Here are some strategies for enhancing your sex life and achieving greater satisfaction:

- **Communicate openly with your partner.** Talk about how you feel, what you want or need from your relationship and how to be intimate in a way that's pleasurable for both of you. If you have unspoken fears regarding sexual contact, such as a fear of pain or a fear of being rejected because of your appearance, tell your partner about them. Talking openly together about your fears can help ease them.

- **Look for ways to rekindle your romance.** Go on a date, plan a picnic, send flowers or exchange personal gifts. To set the stage for sexual intimacy, have dinner by candlelight or hold hands while taking an evening stroll.

- **Prepare your body.** Do gentle range-of-motion exercises for a few minutes before having sex. This may help prevent pain and muscle stiffness. A warm bath or shower with your partner also may help warm and relax your muscles and set the stage for your intimate time. Taking a pain medication or muscle relaxant before sex also may be helpful. Talk with your doctor about which type and dose is right for you.

- **Expand your definition of intimacy.** For many people with arthritis, it's the act of intercourse that causes the most problems. Options that might be more comfortable and fulfilling include cuddling, fondling, sensual massage, masturbation, oral sex or the use of a vibrator.

- **Experiment with different positions that may make intercourse more comfortable.** Instead of the traditional "missionary position," which may be the most painful, try lying side by side, kneeling or sitting. Many good books are available that describe different ways to have intercourse.

- **Make changes to your routine.** Many people often have higher pain levels in the evening. If this is true for you, try being intimate in the morning — when you are refreshed from a good night's sleep and may have the most energy.

If you continue to have sexual problems, talk with your doctor. Describe when and how your sexual desire or performance began to be affected by your arthritis. Pain and fatigue can reduce your libido, but many medications, including glucocorticoids and anti-depressants, also can reduce your sexual drive. Your doctor may be able to change your medication, change the dosage or recommend other strategies to enhance your sex life. One important note: If you suspect a medication may be affecting your sexual performance, don't stop taking it without first consulting your doctor.

In all partnerships, it takes effort to maintain what is good and to correct what isn't. A healthy sexual relationship can positively affect all aspects of your life, including your physical health, self-esteem, productivity and other relationships.

Remind yourself that problems are also opportunities. In your efforts to become more intimate, you may discover something about your partner you otherwise might have missed. The relationship you recover may be even better than the one you had before you developed arthritis.

Simplifying your life

We live in an era of "multitasking" — doing — or trying to do — several things at once. Yet many people seem to long for a simpler, slower-paced, more meaningful life. Although you may not want to quit your job and move to the country, your arthritis may force you to slow down to allow more time for rest and self-care. In addition, you may want to pamper yourself by paying more attention to the things in your life that give you satisfaction and pleasure.

Mayo Clinic psychologist Barbara Bruce, Ph.D., offers these suggestions for simplifying your life:

- **Reassess success.** Living a fast-paced, competitive lifestyle may be exciting at times, but it may not always be the right choice for you. You may make more money, have a better golf score or a high profile in your community, but is it worth the added stress? Making better use of your time and adding more meaning to your life may require giving up some clout to do the things you find truly rewarding. Is your job eating up too many hours of your day? Think about having more time — even if it means less money.

- **Accept the things you can't change.** Maybe you can't do everything you did before you had arthritis. If you have rheumatoid arthritis, the wax-and-wane nature of your disease might make it difficult for you to plan, and you may be too tired to pursue every interest. Don't fight it. Decide what's important and assign priorities. Give those things you both must and want to do top priority. For the rest, delegate them, drop them or ask for help.

- **Take a breath.** When you're rushed or stressed, your breathing is quick and shallow. Relaxed breathing is deep and slow. You can slow down by practicing deep breathing. Inhale slowly to a count of four, then exhale slowly to a count of four. Do this several times a day — whenever you're feeling rushed. Practice deep breathing when you're on hold, waiting in line or working on a deadline. Or let the ring of the telephone signal you to breathe deeply before you answer.

- **Practice saying no.** You can't do everything, especially when you have arthritis. The next time someone asks for your help, think before you say yes. Do you have the time? Are you already overcommitted? Will you have to give up something else you want to do? Is this a project you really want to work on? Are you feeling overwhelmed or worn-out? There's no need to feel guilty. It's OK to say no. Besides, you won't be much use to anyone else if you're running on empty.

- **Own less, clean less.** Unless it's edible, just about everything you bring into your house requires time- and energy-consuming maintenance. Perhaps you once enjoyed your figurine collection, but now you view it as a dust collection. Apply the "pleasure principle" to your possessions. Do they really make you happy? What would you take along if you had to evacuate your home in one hour? Consider getting rid of anything that doesn't significantly add to your life. If you haven't used it in a year, maybe you should put it in storage or give it away. And avoid buying things you don't need.

Learning how to help yourself

The Arthritis Foundation Self-Help Course educates people about the different kinds of arthritis, teaches them how to exercise, explains the appropriate use of arthritis medications and stress management techniques, and encourages participants to take an active role in managing their condition.

Sponsored by the Arthritis Foundation, the educational program was first developed in 1979. Since then it has been proven to reduce arthritis pain by 20 percent and doctor visits by 40 percent. The course has also been shown to decrease depression and increase knowledge about arthritis, exercise, relaxation and self-confidence.

Follow-up studies show that participants tend to make the healthy behavior changes taught in the course, such as exercising. However, improvements in pain, depression and activity level are most closely linked to a positive adjustment in attitude. Course graduates are more confident that they can deal with their disease, as measured by psychological tests. Contact your local Arthritis Foundation chapter for more information about the Arthritis Self-Help Course nearest you.

The rest is rest

Throughout this chapter, you've read about what you can do to gain control over your arthritis and enhance your quality of life. Certainly not the least of these is getting adequate rest. Ours is a sleep-deprived culture in which achievement is often valued over taking care of ourselves. For many, it's a source of pride not to get much sleep. More and more studies are showing the debilitating effects of sleep deprivation for the population in general. But for you, your arthritis makes it imperative that you listen to your body and give it what it needs, especially when it comes to rest.

When should you rest? When you're tired. Arthritis, particularly rheumatoid arthritis, makes you more prone to fatigue. Know your limits. If you need to rest in a comfortable chair or nap during the day, do so. And be sure to get a good night's sleep. Sleep as many hours as you need, not as many as you think you should have. There are no prizes awarded for getting by on four hours a night, despite the culture, and you could aggravate your arthritis by not sleeping enough.

One caveat: It's possible to sleep too much. If you're depressed, you might seek refuge in sleep. Keep naps relatively short, especially if you find them interfering with your sleep at night. As an alternative to a nap, find a comfortable chair and rest without falling asleep. It's OK to be a little tired. And be sure to intersperse rest periods with periods of exercise and other activity.

You're in control

Self-efficacy is a term researchers use. It refers to the belief that you can have control over things that affect your life or that you can master specific situations. Research shows that self-efficacy is the best predictor of positive health outcomes in many situations, including who will cope well with arthritis. Achieving success, such as reducing your stress through one of the relaxation techniques, increases self-efficacy, as does seeing other people succeed in controlling the effects of their illness.

Through the power of your thoughts, feelings and beliefs about your illness and your life, you can help manage arthritis.

Chapter 14

Traveling with arthritis

Travel can be stressful even when you're healthy. But if you have arthritis, the thought of simple activities such as carrying luggage, changing planes or walking long distances can be enough to give you second thoughts about traveling.

But because you have arthritis doesn't mean that you're stuck with a life of immobility. In fact, today it's easier to travel with a disability — either for business or pleasure — than ever before. Laws such as the Americans with Disabilities Act (ADA) and the Air Carrier Access Act have prompted travel suppliers, from airlines to hotels to cruise ships, to make travel easier and more accessible for people who have special needs. In addition, a range of new and established companies have recognized a growing market in serving to clients who have mildly to severely limited abilities, with operators developing special tours, vacation packages and activities for people with arthritis.

Planning your trip

Where in the world do you want to go? Maybe you long to visit the Louvre in Paris or hike the Appalachian Trail in Virginia. Or maybe your company just needs you to solve a problem in Cleveland. The key to any successful trip starts with planning. With the right research, the world is yours for the exploring.

Naturally, you must be honest about your capabilities. Rock climbing might not be the best choice for someone with hip and knee limitations. A mountaintop helicopter excursion, though, might be an alternative. White-water rafting could be extremely painful with a neck condition. A week in a riverside cabin, though, might let you appreciate the water without discomfort.

Choose a vacation that allows you to be flexible. Consider how you'll spend a day alone if your travel companions plan more strenuous activities or extensive sightseeing. Remember, frequent rest periods may be the most important ingredient for a satisfying trip.

Researching your trip is important. You can get a better idea of where you want to travel by preparing carefully. Get information from the places you want to visit. Query tour companies that offer vacations that appeal to you. Read travel guides and visit travel Web sites, including those geared toward people with disabilities.

Should you buy trip insurance?

Although some hotels and airlines will refund your money if you become ill — be sure to send a doctor's statement with your refund request — it's probably best to purchase trip cancellation insurance for expensive trips if you think there's a chance you'll be unable to travel. The policies are available from your travel agent or tour operator. Be aware that charter cancellation insurance may not pay if you cancel because of a preexisting condition.

Review your medical insurance coverage before you go. Policies sometimes include costs of medical illness while you're away from home, including travel back home if you become ill, but many plans don't include this coverage. Some policies exclude preexisting conditions, so be certain to read the fine print. The AAA, formerly known as the American Automobile Association, offers low-cost trip insurance that's available even to nonmembers. The Consumer Reports Travel Letter is a good source of information about this and other travel topics.

Conversations with people who have taken similar trips can help you decide where you want to go and what you can expect when you arrive. And get your doctor's advice when planning a trip. He or she may have a good idea of what you can handle and how you can accomplish your travel goals.

Do you need a professional?

Many people rely on travel agents and tour operators. In most cases agents don't charge for their services, and these professionals can save you time and money. Tour operators generally combine several travel components, such as airline, hotels and ground transportation, into one package that is usually less expensive than what you would pay if you put them together yourself. The fees of tour operators are usually included in these expenses.

To select a travel agent, start by asking friends and relatives for referrals. You can also call agencies and ask about their experience in arranging trips for travelers with physical limitations. Choose an agent with whom you're comfortable discussing your particular needs, and make sure he or she is willing to spend the extra time on your individual arrangements. Treat your agent as a travel partner who wants to work for you after you've made the decisions about what you want and need.

Booking a hotel

Where you sleep at night can make or break a vacation or business trip, so keep your physical needs in mind when choosing lodging. Many large hotel chains publish free directories that describe special accommodations, but be sure to specify what you'll require well in advance. And always get written confirmation of any guaranteed arrangements.

You'll want to ask other things about where you'll be staying. For example, find out how close you'll be to the convention center, restaurant, pool or beach, where the elevators are located, whether bathrooms have handrails, whether the hotel shuttle can be used by someone with physical limitations and whether the doors and faucets have levers instead of hard-to-grasp knobs. Ask whether the hotel has porters to help with luggage and if there's taxicab service if you're going to need it. You may also want to know about the availability of laundry and room services, and about handicapped parking, fire exits and access ramps.

In many cases hotels are equipped to offer a range of special amenities and services, such as tours in accessible vans, heating pads for those unexpected flare-ups or in-house spas with whirlpools. It pays to ask as many questions as possible before you book.

And you're not limited to the major hotel chains either. An increasing number of bed-and-breakfasts, inns and other alternative accommodations now host travelers with disabilities. Most bed-and-breakfast guides include designations to indicate accessible rooms.

What to take along

Remember to pack light. It's good advice for all travelers, but especially for people with arthritis. This means you'll need to plan carefully so that you can satisfy whatever clothing changes you need, plus have all of the important items that make your arthritis more manageable. Don't forget to bring any aids you use daily, such as a raised toilet seat, long-handled reachers, special pillows or a heating pad. If you have electrical appliances or aids and are traveling to a foreign country, you may need to pack a plug or voltage adapter.

Use lightweight luggage with wheels or shoulder straps that make it easier to move. Check to see if porters and taxicabs will be available where you'll need them. Ask porters and taxicab drivers to carry your luggage whenever possible. At the airport, check your bags at the curb. Be sure to carry small bills for tipping people who assist you.

Always check the climate for your destination to decide what type of clothing will be most appropriate. Anything that can be layered lets you adapt easily to weather changes. In most cases loose clothing that allows maximal freedom of movement is best.

Packing tips

- Pack as little as possible. Lay out the essentials, then leave half of them at home.
- Use lightweight luggage with sturdy wheels, a telescoping handle and a shoulder strap. This gives you maximum flexibility. Even if you don't take the baggage with you into the passenger compartment, carry-on luggage with wheels is practical and lightweight and can help you limit the amount of things you take along.
- Bring a pillow if you have neck problems. You can buy small ones that fit inside your luggage, or roll up a towel to fit your neck and tape the loose end.
- Lotion, oils and menthol gels are great for quick self-massages between sightseeing activities.
- Most U.S. airlines allow just one or two carry-on bags.
- Airlines allow two pieces of checked luggage. Medical equipment, such as wheelchairs, spare batteries, battery chargers and necessary supplies, isn't included in the limit and is transported at no extra charge. Just be sure that bags or boxes contain medical supplies and nothing else.

Sunscreen, sunglasses, a wide-brimmed hat and comfortable shoes also are essential.

When packing medications, take more than enough to last through your trip, and carry them in their original containers. It's best to transport medicines in your carry-on luggage in case you're separated from the bags you've checked, although some travelers pack duplicates in their luggage. If you need medications kept cool, most train and airline personnel will gladly put them in the refrigerator, although you may prefer to carry them in a vacuum flask or insulated container.

Along with your medications, bring copies of your prescriptions, your doctor's name and telephone and fax numbers, a summary of your medical history and a list of your medications. It's a good idea to leave a copy of this information at home with a friend or relative in case your doctor is unavailable. You also might consider wearing a medical alert bracelet or necklace if you have other medical problems in addition to arthritis.

Traveling by air

With passage of the Air Carrier Access Act, U.S. airlines and terminals have become more accommodating. After the 1986 ruling, the Department of Transportation developed new regulations that outlaw discrimination against disabled travelers by describing the responsibilities of travelers, carriers, airport operators and contractors. For people with arthritis, the rules mean more time for boarding, accessible terminal parking and accessible restrooms, among other things.

Still, you must do your part. When you make airline reservations, always remember to state special needs, such as diet, seating or storage capacity for oversized arthritis aids. Allow extra time to get through the airport, request an airport wheelchair or other terminal transport if you need it and check your luggage through to your final destination.

If you feel you've experienced a disability-related service problem, you may call a toll-free Department of Transportation (DOT) hotline to report the problem. The number is (800) 778-4838, and it's staffed between 7 a.m. and 11 p.m. Eastern Time seven days a week. If you want the DOT to investigate the problem, you must submit a complaint in writing

Security at all airports in the United States with scheduled airline service requires that passengers go through a preboarding screening process. The Transportation Security Administration (TSA) has several suggestions for people with disabilities and medical conditions to help make the screening process go smoothly. Those suggestions include:

- If you need assistance moving through the airport, contact your airline. Your airline can provide someone to assist you through the airport and the screening line.
- If you require a companion or assistant to accompany you through the security checkpoint to reach the boarding gate,

contact your airline about getting a gate pass for your companion. Do this before reaching the security checkpoint.

- The limit of one carry-on and one personal item (purse, briefcase, computer case) doesn't apply to medical supplies, equipment, mobility aids or assistive devices that you require.
- Pack medications in a separate bag to help speed the inspection process. Make sure the medication container isn't too densely filled and that it's clearly labeled.
- If you have medical documentation of your condition or disability, you may present this information to the screener to help inform him or her. Such documentation isn't required and having it won't exempt you from the screening process. In addition, tell the screener about any special equipment or devices that you're using or about any devices located in or on your body.
- Make sure that all your carry-on items, equipment, mobility aids and assistive devices have an identification tag attached.
- Several items, including wheelchairs, scooters, crutches, canes, walkers, prosthetic devices, braces and orthopedic shoes, are permitted through the security checkpoint.
- If you have tools required to remove a prosthetic device, the TSA recommends that you bring them along should you need to remove the prosthesis for any reason.
- If you have a medical device either inside or outside of your body, check with your doctor to learn if it's safe for you to go through a metal detector or to be handwanded. If your doctor says that it's not safe, then ask the screener for a pat-down inspection instead.
- If a personal search is required, you may request a private area for screening. You may request a private area at any time during the screening process.
- Ask the screener for assistance if you need help as you proceed through the screening, including walking through the metal detector.

Certain times of the day are less congested for airlines, making travel easier to negotiate. Reservationists also can recommend less crowded flights. If you must change planes, find out whether you also need to change terminals. If so, ask whether a shuttle between them is accessible. If not, ask for suggestions on making the move.

Traveling by train

Trains generally provide a good transportation option. Throughout Europe, rail travel is easy and accessible, with Eurostar trains accommodating disabled travelers on international routes. In the United States, Amtrak offers special assistance and reduced fares for disabled passengers.

When making Amtrak reservations, request accessible seating, assisted boarding and special meals. Most train stations have personnel to provide baggage assistance and to help get passengers from the station entrance onto the train. Amtrak suggests that you make requests for assistance when you make your reservations.

Sister Gertrude's wheels

My three-wheeled Amigo, a battery-powered wheelchair, can't go more than 5 mph. But in France, a police officer pulled me over for speeding one September day.

I was on my way back to the hotel, after worshipping in Our Lady of Lourdes, a church built in a valley of the Pyrenees mountains to commemorate the Virgin Mary's appearance in 1858. Pilgrims go there for healing of body and soul. Rain pelted us as we left the church, and I was afraid that the water might damage my Amigo. So I was in a hurry to get back to the hotel, a half-mile away. But rolling along slowly in front of me was a long string of wheelchairs, perhaps 20 or more. So I pulled out into the road to pass them. That's when the police officer raised his hand and took out his ticket pad. He looked serious.

I guess I was supposed to follow the other wheelchairs without passing. Fortunately, some French-speaking lady in my travel group talked to the police officer. I don't know what she said, but it made him smile and he waved me on, without a ticket.

If you have trouble walking, Amtrak can supply a wheelchair. If you have your own wheelchair, it must conform to the ADA definition of a "common" wheelchair. That is, the chair must not exceed 30 inches in width, 48 inches in length, 2 inches in ground clearance and weigh no more than 600 pounds occupied. Most stations have wheelchair lifts.

Traveling by bus

Many bus lines have terminals with convenient restrooms, wide doorways and handrails. Most bus aisles, however, aren't wide enough for wheelchairs. If you use a wheelchair or have trouble using stairs, make arrangements with customer service for assistance in getting on and off the bus at your point of departure and your destination.

Months earlier, when I told my friends that I was going to Lourdes to fulfill a longtime dream, they said it was impossible. I was 73 years old. Damage from osteoarthritis had required me to have a knee replacement. I wore braces on my knees, back and neck. And I needed my Amigo to travel more than a few yards. But I found a tour company that specializes in trips for disabled people. And I got travel tips from many sources, such as the Arthritis Foundation, Mayo Clinic and the makers of my wheelchair.

On my Amigo I roamed airports and traveled the curb-cut streets of Lourdes, stopping at sidewalk cafes and, once, climbing a steep hill to a chapel. I even took a three-day side trip to Paris on a six-hour train ride through the beautiful countryside.

There were a few surprises, such as bus lifts that didn't always work. But I was determined to enjoy myself. And I did.

Sister Gertrude Ann
Rochester, Minn.

Because bus travel is often slower, you may want to schedule trips in midweek when fewer people travel. In addition, avoid trips with many transfers. Take along a pillow and snacks, such as fresh fruits, raw vegetables, no-salt crackers and peanut butter or low-fat cheese. Keep your medications and bottled water with you.

Traveling by car

When you travel by car, you'll enjoy more freedom than with any other form of transportation. You can stop whenever you want, you'll have more room to stretch out, and you can take along anything that will fit in your vehicle.

And there are ways to make the trip even more enjoyable. Be sure to stop as often as feasible, getting out to stretch and move around. Keep medications, snacks, maps, emergency kit and first-aid supplies in the car, and consider taking along a cellular phone. Your cell phone may not work overseas, but you can usually rent one at your destination. Make hotel or motel reservations in advance, or stop early enough to find a place to stay. Don't let yourself become overtired before finding a bed for the night.

When renting a car, ask for amenities that will make driving more comfortable, such as hand controls, a transfer board if you use a wheelchair, swivel seats and a spinner knob for the steering wheel. To get a car with special features, you generally need to reserve your vehicle 48 hours in advance.

Traveling by ship

You may find cruise travel particularly relaxing. Substantial design changes have been made to U.S. flagships in recent years, such as widening of passageways, doorways and elevators, and accessible staterooms for wheelchair travelers have been added. Special diets and exercise plans may be available, too.

The United States Supreme Court in 2005 ruled that cruise ships must follow federal law that bars discrimination against disabled people. The Supreme Court left it to lower courts to decide exactly what changes would have to be adopted by foreign flagships operating in U.S. waters. So be sure to check before booking to make sure the cruise you're planning will have the accommodations that you need. Before booking with a particular cruise line, ask plenty of questions about the ship's design and accessibility. You'll want to book a cabin as close to the action as possible, but you'll need to decide if that means proximity to restaurants, pools or sundecks.

If you anticipate difficulty in embarking or disembarking, choose a cruise with fewer stops, or plan to stay on board soaking up the ship's ambience when others have gone ashore. Choices abound these days in cruises geared for the more leisurely traveler, and many shore excursions now accommodate those with an unhurried pace. Most ships employ doctors, but their pharmacies are usually limited. You'll want to take along more than enough medication to get you through the trip.

Touring overseas

Most countries have specific services designed for travelers who need special assistance. Whether you're touring Australia or Italy, Venezuela or Singapore, travel professionals are available to help make your trip easier and more comfortable. Many have brochures, toll-free phone numbers and Internet sites where you can find out more about what's offered in each country on your itinerary.

In addition, the International Association for Medical Assistance to Travelers offers a free information packet detailing its services, which include free climate and sanitation information and advice on international disease and immunization requirements. Travel Assistance International provides 24-hour medical referrals to travelers more than 100 miles from home.

Although health care has improved in many world destinations, be sure you're carrying ample medications on overseas trips and pace yourself so that you won't need a doctor to attend a routine flare-up or other short-term condition.

No matter where you're headed, whether it's New England or New Zealand, take all reasonable precautions to ensure your safety, health and well-being. Then relax and have fun. You can travel — and travel well — with arthritis.

Chapter 15

On the job with arthritis

rthritis is no reason to start planning an early retirement. With a positive attitude — focusing on what you can do instead of what you can't — you'll begin discovering creative solutions to the demands you face in the workplace. But your success at the job will depend greatly on having an upbeat attitude, a strong belief that you can and the will to get on with your life.

One of the first challenges you face is whether to tell your boss and your co-workers about your arthritis. Many people are afraid to do this. And with good reason. In some cases arthritis raises questions in your employer's mind about whether you're physically able to do the job. Some who don't understand that arthritis is more than just aches and pains may also wonder whether you're using the disease as an excuse for special treatment. And in some job situations, unspoken discrimination will show up as denied opportunities, such as promotions you earn and deserve but don't get.

For reasons such as these, many experts recommend that you say nothing about the disease if you can answer no to the following questions:

- Is your arthritis obvious?
- Do you need special accommodations or resources to do the job?

If you answer yes to one of these questions, it's usually best to tell your employer and co-workers that you have arthritis. Otherwise, they may grow to believe you aren't carrying your share of the load — and they may resent you for it. If you say nothing and try to keep the arthritis a secret, you'll probably try to overcome the hard feelings of your colleagues by ignoring your body's warning signs and pushing yourself beyond your limits. This will only make matters worse by increasing the pain and fatigue so common to arthritis.

If you decide you need to tell your boss about the your illness, schedule a meeting with care. Pick a time of the day and week when distractions and job pressures for both of you are lower than usual. Then explain that you have arthritis. Give your boss a short course about the disease. If you have rheumatoid arthritis, you might explain that when the pain flares up or fatigue sets in, these are signs that the tissues around your affected joints need rest and repair.

Go into this meeting with suggestions about changes that will help you do a better job. You'll need to do a little research to come up with these ideas. Talk with your doctor or an occupational therapist about your work responsibilities. They'll likely have ideas to help you perform certain tasks more easily, perhaps with the aid of assistive devices — such as armrests on your chair — or with exercises that will increase your dexterity and range of motion for any repeated movements you'll have to do during your workday.

Your rights

The Americans with Disabilities Act passed by Congress in 1990. It is the most extensive bill of rights for people with disabilities ever signed into law.

This law bans discrimination against people with disabilities, and it requires companies with 15 or more employees to make reasonable changes to help individuals do their jobs. In fact, wise employers will value your experience and will be willing to give you the tools necessary for you to do your job well. Among the possible reasonable accommodations are the following:

- Providing or modifying equipment to help you perform your job tasks, such as a wheeled cart to carry supplies, a headphone instead of a handheld receiver or a chair with good back support. The cost of some assistive devices may qualify your employer for tax benefits.
- Providing a ramp if you have difficulty with stairs. If accommodations or special equipment is required, the employer cannot make you pay for it. An exception would be if the changes place an undue hardship on the employer, causing significant expense or difficulty. What constitutes undue hardship is a matter judged on a case-by-case basis.
- Adjusting the height of your desk.
- Allowing break periods for rest.
- Changing your job responsibilities, eliminating tasks you can't perform that are not essential to your job.

If you believe your employer treats you unfairly and is unwilling to make reasonable changes to help you do your job, you can file a formal complaint with the Equal Employment Opportunity Commission (EEOC). Free brochures about the Americans with Disabilities Act are available from the EEOC. Your state also may have laws to protect you from discrimination. If you have questions about your legal rights, you may also wish to speak with a lawyer who specializes in employment law.

Protect your joints

Finding ways to reduce or eliminate activities that irritate, inflame or damage your joints can keep you off disability and in the workforce longer. Here are some suggestions to keep in mind as you plan:

- Arrange your office or work area to reduce the amount of lifting, walking or other movement that may be painful.
- Find the most comfortable position for doing your work.
- If you perform repetitive motions, such as typing or assembly work, rest the affected joints every 20 to 30 minutes by stretching your muscles. In fact, even if you don't perform repetitive

motions, try to take a short break every half-hour or hour. Change positions, stretch and relax for a minute or two.

- If one particular task is always painful, search for other ways to do it. Occupational therapists specialize in solving such problems. Another option might be to ask a co-worker to help you out in exchange for your help on something else.
- Use special tools or assistive devices that reduce strain on your joints: electric staplers, dictation services, chair-leg extensions (to make it easier to get up) and enlarged grips for pencils and pens.

Exercise

Maintaining the muscle strength around your joints helps keep the joints stable and more comfortable. Your doctor and your physical therapist can design an exercise program that allows you to work on the joints that you use most often in your job. Some of the exercises can be simple and inconspicuous enough that you can do them at lunch or during momentary breaks. For example, if you work a lot with your hands, you can take a few seconds to bend your fingers, wrists and elbows as far as you can, then stretch them back out.

Relax

Job stress can aggravate arthritic pain, which intensifies the job stress. One way to break this cycle is to learn relaxation techniques. Following are a few ideas:

- Let your mind wander to a happy memory.
- Look out a window and study a pleasant scene.
- Listen to music or a tape of relaxing sounds, such as the ocean surf or a gentle rain.
- Sit outside or take a short walk.
- Lie down or sit quietly for a few minutes and, with eyes closed, practice deep breathing. Then, starting with your toes, tighten the muscles and then release them. Work your way up to your scalp, then let your mind and body slip into a minute of relaxation. Avoid if tensing your muscles aggravates your arthritis.

Conserve your energy

Arthritis can cause fatigue. You can help avoid fatigue by pacing yourself and by doing the most important projects during your time of peak energy. For example, if you're a morning person and you do various tasks throughout the day, spend the morning doing the work that requires the most concentration and energy. In addition, schedule working breathers by alternating difficult tasks with easier ones. If possible, take a rest break of about 10 minutes every few hours.

Be a smart commuter

For some with arthritis, the trip to work can become a painful and exhausting gauntlet of obstacles: stress-inducing traffic, driving a vehicle that isn't equipped for people with restricted movement, then walking from the company's distant parking lot and up a flight of stairs. Each one of these can cause a flare-up of arthritic pain and can sap your energy before the workday begins. Try these ideas:

- Share a ride with someone who works with you or in your area. Pay for the service or take turns driving.
- Use public transportation. It's usually slower but is less exhausting than driving in bumper-to-bumper traffic. The Americans with Disabilities Act requires accessible public transit vehicles be available to individuals with disabilities.
- If you must drive, install equipment that will minimize the discomfort: backrest, special mirrors, steering wheel modifications. Some automakers give you rebates when you install these kinds of equipment in new cars, and they'll give you a list of companies in your area that will do the installation.
- If you have trouble walking, ask your employer for a parking space near the entrance. You can get a parking decal for the disabled by contacting your state transportation department. This allows you to use parking spaces reserved for the handicapped.
- If you have difficulty with stairs, you may need to ask for a ramp leading into the building. You might also request a work space near the entrance.

Make friends with your computer

Working at a keyboard for the better part of eight hours a day can worsen the pain and fatigue of arthritis. If you work at a computer, consider these tips:

- As you sit in your chair, lean back slightly so that your lower back is against the backrest. Keep your feet flat on the floor, with your knees bent at about 90 degrees or slightly more. If you have no firm lumbar support, ask for a chair that allows you to adjust the backrest to different heights and angles.
- Move up close to the keyboard, so you aren't reaching out at it. The keyboard should be about 3 to 6 inches from your lap. Both the keyboard and the monitor should be directly in front of you. The top of the monitor screen should be at eye level.
- A wrist rest, or padded bar, between the keyboard and your lap provides wrist support by giving your hands a place to rest as you type. While typing, your wrists should be straight, with your forearms parallel to the floor. Wrist braces can help keep your wrists in the proper position. And chairs with armrests offer support for the forearms. If your wrists are usually bent as you type and have no support, you can develop carpal tunnel syndrome. This produces pain or numbness in your hands, which can radiate to your arms.
- If typing is difficult for you, use a mouse as much as possible. Another option is voice activation software. This allows you to dictate to the computer, which types the words as you speak.
- Take short breaks from the computer to stretch your legs, arms and fingers. Give your eyes a break by focusing on something at a distance, such as an object out the window or across the room.

Keep an open mind about your job and career

Despite all that you and your employer can do to accommodate for your arthritis, the nature of your job or the progression of your arthritis may require you to cut back on the number of hours you work or to find another line of work.

If your job requires heavy physical labor, such as construction, your doctor may refer you to an occupational therapist or to a vocational rehabilitation agency to build your strength and to determine how much weight you can safely lift. If the restrictions are such that there's no job you can do in the company, the vocational rehabilitation agency can help you find a job that you can do. Sometimes, workers decide to join a related company. A construction worker, for example, may join an business that sells equipment for the construction industry.

Some job hunting tips

Although employers aren't allowed to ask if you have a disability, they may ask if you're able to perform specific job functions. A sample question might be: "Do you have any physical limitations that would hinder your performance in the job that you're applying for?" Such questions can put you in an awkward situation if you think you'll need some kind of assistance in doing the work.

Some career counselors say that during the initial interview you shouldn't disclose that you have arthritis. They suggest that doing so could eliminate you as a candidate without giving you a chance to discuss the matter. For this reason, they suggest answering no, under the presumption that the employer will provide the legally required reasonable accommodations if this becomes necessary. Another possible response if you're not sure how your arthritis will affect your job performance is to write "Will discuss" on the application.

If your arthritis will be obvious to the interviewer, consider dropping a hint about it during the set-up phone conversation — but only after you make the interview appointment, and only if the person you're talking to is the one who will be interviewing you. Possible hint: "I sometimes have trouble with stairs. Do you have an elevator?" Hints like this may help reduce the shock, making it easier for the interviewer to concentrate on your discussion.

Perhaps the most popular interview question is, "Tell me about yourself." As friendly as this may seem, this type of open-ended question is not a pleasant icebreaker. It has the potential to be the

most dangerous question of the day for you — or the most beneficial. Law prohibits employers from basing their hiring decisions on
age, sex, race, religion, health or nonfelony arrests. They aren't supposed to ask, "How's your health?" But in describing yourself, you
may reveal the answer. If you plan you can answer the question
well and avoid revealing the "illegal" information, unless you want
to do so.

Briefly summarize assets you would bring to the job. For example, you could say that you place a high value on education, earned
a college degree in your chosen career and were fortunate enough
to have had two excellent jobs in the field. You could add that your
experience, your desire to excel and your eagerness to accept new
challenges have led you here.

If your arthritis is obvious, you may want to mention it briefly
during the interview. But don't shift the focus to your limitations.
Talk about adjustments you've made that allow you to stay productive. For instance, you could say something like this: "I know
you're legally prohibited from asking about my arthritis, except
questions about how I would do specific tasks required on the job.
But I'd be happy to answer any questions you have because I'm
certain I can do the work."

If your arthritis isn't obvious but will require job accommodations, you face a tough dilemma that has no easy solution. Should
you say nothing until you have a job offer? If so, you can be certain
that you won't be ruled out because of your disability. But the
employer might feel misled. And this could generate hard feelings
and a shaky start to your new job. Another approach is to tell the
employer about your arthritis, especially if you know there are
areas in which you'll need some accommodation very soon.
Employers aren't obligated to provide accommodations until you
tell them that you have a disability. If you decide this is the best
solution for you, mention that the accommodations are usually
inexpensive and well worth the investment.

With a positive outlook and thoughtful preparation, you have
every right to be hopeful about your future in the workplace.

Chapter 16

Where to get more help

Here are selected sources, plus some general recommendations on how to search for arthritis information.

The Arthritis Foundation

The Arthritis Foundation is an excellent source of information and support. This national organization works mainly through state and regional chapters. It offers self-help materials, support groups, exercise and water aerobics classes, and lists of doctors in your area who are experienced in working with people who have arthritis.

The business white pages of the telephone book lists local Arthritis Foundation chapters. To order informational brochures, subscribe to the magazine *Arthritis Today* or learn how to contact your local chapter, call the Arthritis Foundation at (800) 568-4045. The Arthritis Foundation's address is P.O. Box 7669, Atlanta, GA 30357. The telephone number of the national office is (404) 872-7100. Many countries outside the United States — including Canada, Australia and New Zealand — have similar organizations. The telephone number of the national office of the Canadian Arthritis Society is (416) 979-7228.

Mayo Clinic health information

Mayo Clinic offers numerous resources for reliable health information. Mayo Clinic's Health Information Web site at *www.MayoClinic.com* provides timely, accurate information on many health topics, including arthritis. To access information on arthritis from the home page, look for "Disease and Condition Centers" and then click "Arthritis."

From time to time, the monthly publications *Mayo Clinic Health Letter* and *Mayo Clinic Women's HealthSource* contain information about recent developments in arthritis treatment.

Surfing the Web

If you have a personal computer and Internet access, you can find a lot of information on the Web. The Food and Drug Administration (FDA) and many other government agencies, private organizations, groups and individuals use the Web to offer in-depth information. Here are some of the better Web sites for locating reliable information about arthritis:

- The Arthritis Foundation Web site at *www.arthritis.org*.
- The Department of Health and Human Services Web site at *www.healthfinder.gov*. The site offers links to the Web sites of clearinghouses, databases, support groups and government agencies. Go to the home page, click "Health Library" and select "Diseases and Conditions." You'll find an alphabetical list that includes "Arthritis."
- Use government information on the Web to compare the benefits of managed care health insurance plans offered in your area. A government Medicare site provides comparative information at *www.medicare.gov/mphCompare/home.asp*. Search this information by state or Zip code. View benefits for a single plan or directly compare the benefits of two separate plans.
- The National Institute of Arthritis and Musculoskeletal and Skin Diseases (NIAMS), part of the National Institutes of Health, at *www.niams.nih.gov/hi*.

- The American Medical Association and several other medical associations have a Web site that includes information on health conditions. To access arthritis information, go to *www.medem.com,* click "Medem Medical Library,"then "Diseases and Conditions," and "Bone, Joint and Rheumatic Conditions."
- The American College of Rheumatology at *www.rheumatology.org.* You can access arthritis information and the latest press releases from the home page.

Your local library

Become familiar with the resources available at your public library. Reference areas routinely stock medical dictionaries, and the periodical section may carry the monthly *Arthritis Today.* Find out which books about arthritis are on the shelves. If you're considering purchasing costly equipment, check the consumer information section. Today's technology makes libraries the source of information from around the world. Ask the reference librarian about the best way to search for information you need. If you don't own a computer, your library may have one you can use at no charge.

Words of caution

The Web is a source of seemingly endless medical information, some of it very good, but some of it downright bad medical advice. Don't believe everything you read on the Web. Anyone who has the necessary hardware and software can publish a health information Web page or offer medical advice in an online chat forum. And the Internet has a way of making all health information appear equal. Be particularly wary of products offered for sale online.

Stick with reliable sources for your medical advice. Before you delve too far into a radical new treatment, whether on the Web or elsewhere, determine who's sponsoring it. Is the sponsor qualified to give medical advice or sell something? Is the information updated frequently? Is it reviewed by health care professionals?

Buyer beware

Each year one in four Americans uses quack medical treatments, collectively spending at least $27 billion for these treatments. At best, the drugs, devices and lifestyle changes are worthless. At worst, they may lead to physical harm and even death. Medical quackery succeeds because people yearn for a quick cure.

The American Medical Association estimates that most victims of fraudulent medical treatments spend $500 to $1,000 annually. But beyond being useless and expensive, sometimes fraudulent medical treatments are actually dangerous. Medications, even vitamins, that are harmless when taken in moderation may be very dangerous when taken in doses prescribed by the quack.

Watch out for promotions that describe medical treatments with adjectives such as *secret, proven, miracle, foreign, breakthrough* and *overnight*. Also be wary of glowing testimonials. Quacks tend to claim they're fighting against a conspiracy of established physicians who are unwilling to acknowledge new treatments. They claim their products provide a complete cure without any side effects. And they often exert pressure, claiming that this is a "limited offer," available for only a short time. At this time, there is no cure for arthritis. But there are many ways to have a positive impact on your health.

Ask whether newspaper or magazine articles attribute the information to a respected publication, organization or medical professional. Carefully examine statistics. It typically takes years of consecutive studies to prove cause and effect. Read reports about medical studies carefully and check sources. Did the study involve a large number of people? Was there a control group? Do the results show a cause-and-effect relationship or an association between two factors? Has the work been published in a peer-reviewed medical journal? If something you find sounds questionable or conflicts with conventional wisdom, be skeptical. If health news makes you question your treatment, medication or diet, ask your doctor whether the information applies to you.

Equipment resources

Mayo Clinic Store
200 1st Street S.W.
Siebens Building Subway Level
Rochester, MN 55905
(507) 284-9669 or (988) 303-9354
www.mayoclinic.org/mayo-store
(order free catalog online)

AliMed
297 High Street
Dedham, MA 02026
(800) 225-2610
www.alimed.com

Anderson Wheel Chair &
Therapeutic Supply
1117 Second St. S.W.
Rochester, MN 55902
(507) 288-0113 or (800) 253-2770

Sammons Preston Rolyan
270 Remington Blvd., Suite C
Bolingbrook, IL 60440
(800) 323-5547
www.sammonspreston.com

Aids for Arthritis
35 Wakefield Drive
Medford, NJ 08055
(800) 654-0707
www.aidsforarthritis.com

Sears Home Health and
Wellness Catalog
7700 Brush Hill Road, Suite 240
Burr Ridge, IL 60527

National headquarters:
Arthritis Foundation
P.O. Box 7669
Atlanta, GA 30357
(800) 283-7800
www.arthritis.org

Assistive devices

ABLEDATA
8630 Fenton St., Suite 930
Silver Spring, MD 20910
(800) 227-0216
www.abledata.com

Job Accommodation Network
P.O. Box 6080
Morgantown, WV 26506
(304) 293-7186 or (800) 526-7234
www.jan.wvu.edu

Office of Disability
Employment Policy (ODEP)
U.S. Department of Labor
200 Constitution Ave., N.W.
Washington, D.C. 20210
(866) 633-7365
www.dol.gov/odep

National Rehabilitation
Information Center
4200 Forbes Blvd.
Suite 202
Lanham, MD 20706
(800) 346-2742
www.naric.com

American Occupational
Therapy Association
4720 Montgomery Lane
P.O. Box 31220
Bethesda, MD 20824-1220
(301) 652-2682 or (800) 729-2682
www.aota.org

Department of Justice
Civil Rights Division
950 Pennsylvania Ave. N.W.
Washington, D.C. 20530
www.usdoj.gov/crt

American Bar Association
321 N. Clark St.
Chicago, IL 60610
(800) 285-2221
www.abanet.org

Legal issues

U.S. Equal Employment
Opportunity Commission
(202) 663-4900 or (800) 669-4000
www.eeoc.gov/publications.html
Free brochures — "The ADA:
Questions and Answers" and
"The ADA: Your Employment
Rights as an Individual With a
Disability" (available online)

Americans With
Disabilities Act
Information Line
(800) 514-0301

Glossary

acupuncture. The practice of piercing specific sites on the body, called pathways or meridians, with thin needles in an attempt to relieve pain associated with some chronic disorders.

acute-phase response. A physiological reaction that occurs after tissue damage. It may include fever, endocrine changes, changes in fluid and electrolyte balance and the synthesis of specific proteins in the blood. An elevated erythrocyte sedimentation rate and elevated C-reactive protein are markers for the presence of an acute phase reaction. The acute phase response helps the body in repairing injured tissue and in defending itself against infection or other disease.

amyloid. A fibrous protein-carbohydrate that's deposited in some tissues during certain chronic diseases, including amyloidosis, rheumatoid arthritis, tuberculosis and Alzheimer's disease. The deposited amyloid interferes with normal tissue function.

anesthesiologist. A doctor who is often involved in treating the pain of arthritis through the use of nerve blocks.

angiogenesis (an-je-o-JEN-uh-sis). The growth of new blood vessels in tissues allowing cells to receive nutrients.

angiography. The X-ray depiction of blood vessels following introduction of contrast material into the bloodstream. Used as a tool to diagnose diseases that affect the blood vessels, including inflammatory diseases.

antibody. A globulin protein produced by the blood that selectively reacts with the protein (antigen) that stimulated its development. In autoimmune disease, antibodies may react with the body's own tissues.

antigen. Any substance capable of inducing an immune response resulting in production of a specific antibody or sensitized lymphocyte that interacts with the antigen. In some autoimmune and arthritic diseases, the body's own tissues may act as antigens.

antinuclear antibodies. The antibodies that interact with cell nuclei. Commonly found in certain autoimmune diseases, including arthritis.

apheresis. A procedure in which blood is collected from a donor with a special machine. Part of the blood, such as platelets or white blood cells, is removed from the blood, and the rest is returned to the donor. Also called pheresis.

arthrodesis (ahrthro-DEE-sis). The surgical fusion of a joint so that the bones grow solidly together, immobilizing the joint. Surgical joint fusion is used to reduce pain and improve stability in the spine, wrist, ankle, feet and other parts of the body.

arthroplasty. Joint surgery done to improve function. May involve insertion of metal alloy or high-density plastic materials or total joint replacement.

arthrocentesis. A procedure using a needle to puncture and withdraw (aspirate) fluid from a joint for medical tests to help with diagnosis. May also be used to inject medication into a joint.

arthroscopy. An examination of the interior of a joint with a small camera mounted in the tip of a tube that's inserted into the joint through a small incision in the skin. The instrument is called an arthroscope.

autoimmune disease. A condition in which the body's immune system reacts against its own tissues. This process is thought to occur in rheumatoid arthritis and some related diseases.

avascular necrosis. A disease resulting from temporary or permanent loss of blood supply to bones. This can lead to tiny breaks within the bone, and can eventually cause bones to collapse.

B-lymphocytes (B-cells). Lymphocytes formed in the bone marrow. They function in immunity related to antibodies (humoral immunity). B-lymphocytes have sites (receptors) on their surfaces where particular antigens can attach. When a B-lymphocyte encounters its specific antigen and it attaches to the receptor, the B-lymphocyte is stimulated to change into a plasma cell which produces antibodies against the antigen. (See also lymphocytes.)

biopsy. The removal of a sample of body tissue for examination — usually microscopic — to aid in diagnosis. A biopsy of a joint may help diagnose an unusual form of arthritis.

bursa. A sac or saclike cavity filled with synovial fluid and situated to reduce friction between moving body tissues, such as a tendon sliding over bone.

carpal tunnel syndrome. A painful and often progressive condition caused by compression of the median nerve in the front part of the wrist. The condition can cause pain, tingling, numbness and weakness in your fingers and thumbs.

cartilage. A fibrous connective tissue. Found in the lining of joints and in the flexible portions of the nose and the ears.

chemokines. Molecules that play a central role in inflammatory responses and trigger migration and activation of phagocytic cells and lymphocytes. Chemokines attract cells of the immune system. Overproduction of chemokines contributes to inflammation, which occurs in autoimmune diseases. For example, overproduction of chemokines in the joints of people with rheumatoid arthritis may lead to invasion of the joint space by destructive immune system cells such as macrophages, neutrophils and T-cells.

chiropractic. Chiropractic treatment is based on the philosophy that restricted movement in the spine or "abnormal alignment" may lead to pain and reduced function of the nervous system and other organs. Spinal adjustment (manipulation) is one form of therapy chiropractors use to treat restricted spinal mobility. The goal is to restore spinal movement and position and, as a result, improve function and decrease pain.

chondrocalcinosis. The calcification of cartilage in a joint due to the accumulation of calcium salt crystals (calcium pyrophosphate dihydrate). Release of the calcium salt crystals into the joint cavity can cause pain, redness, heat and swelling in the joint. These attacks are also referred to as pseudogout.

chondrocytes. Mature cartilage cells that synthesize the structural components and other substances that form and maintain cartilage.

clinical trials. Carefully planned studies that evaluate the benefits and risks of diagnostic tests or treatments in humans. Some clinical trials are also called controlled research trials or double blind studies when conducted in certain ways. Clinical trials help establish the safety and effectiveness of new tests, drugs or treatments.

collagen. A long protein fiber that connects and strengthens various tissues.

complement system. A complex series of proteins that interact with antigen-antibody complexes that are involved in immune and inflammatory reactions. Complement reactions occur in rheumatoid arthritis and lupus erythematosus.

computerized tomography (CT). A method of displaying cross-sections of the body, including joints and the spine, that uses a sequential series of X-rays.

connective tissue disease. Term used for a group of disorders involving one or more of the elements of connective tissue, including collagen, elastin or the mucopolysaccharides. Some connective tissue diseases are inflammatory, such as systemic lupus erythematosus, rheumatoid arthritis, scleroderma and polymyositis. When manifestations of more than one disease are present, the term *mixed connective tissue disease* is sometimes used. Another large but uncommon group of diseases in this category is characterized by inherited defects in connective tissue that results in weakness of the affected tissues. Diseases with these characteristics include Ehlers-Danlos syndrome, Marfan syndrome and xanthoma pseudoelasticum.

crystal-induced arthritis. A form of arthritis (usually acute) set off by release of microcrystals in a joint. The crystals initiate an intense acute inflammatory response. Gout and pseudogout are the two most common forms of crystal-induced arthritis.

cyclooxygenases (COX). These enzymes are involved in the production of prostaglandins, hormonelike substances that trigger inflammation. COX-1 is involved in maintaining normal body functions. COX-2 is more involved in inflammatory reactions.

cyst. A closed cavity or sac in the body.

cytokines. Proteins released by cells that direct cell actions. There are numerous types and sources of cytokines. Similar substances are named lymphokines and interleukins and are prominently involved in inflammation.

dendritic cells. An immune system cell with numerous branching processes. Dendritic cells function by processing antigens or presenting them to T-cells, thereby stimulating cellular immunity.

elastin. A type of connective fiber that is flexible and elastic in various tissues. Helps hold tissues in place.

endothelium. A layer of cells that lines cavities of the body, such as inside joints and blood vessels.

enthesis. The site of attachment of muscle or ligament to bone.

enzymes. Complex proteins produced by cells and that encourage or catalyze a specific biochemical reaction at body temperatures. Our bodies couldn't function without enzymes.

eosinophils. A type of white blood cell containing granules that stain with the dye eosin. Eosinophils are associated with allergic conditions.

epidemiology. The study of the causes of diseases, such as arthritis, by determining their frequencies and relationships to events in the environment.

fibroblasts. Cells in connective tissues that make collagen. Fibroblasts are found in most tissues and form supporting structures for our organs.

frozen shoulder. A painful limitation of motion of the shoulder resulting from chronic inflammation of the rotator cuff.

glucocorticoids. Hormones released from the adrenal glands that affect carbohydrate metabolism. Examples include cortisone and prednisone, which have powerful anti-inflammatory actions but also adverse side effects.

Heberden's nodes. Small, bony nodules found in the fingertip (distal) joints in osteoarthritis.

hemochromatosis. A genetic disorder that causes the body to absorb and store too much iron. The extra iron builds up in organs and damages them. Without treatment, the disease can cause these organs to fail.

human leukocyte antigens (HLA). Proteins determined by inheritance that influence the body's immune system function. Certain types are associated with diseases such as rheumatoid arthritis.

hyaluronic acid. A protein found in large amounts in synovial fluid of joints. It may be altered in arthritis. (*See also* synovial fluid.)

immune complex. The combination of an antigen and antibody. Immune complexes may interact with proteins such as the complement system and produce inflammation and tissue injury. (*See also* complement system.)

immune system. The cells and tissues that protect the body against infection. Disordered immune system function has been associated with the development of arthritis and other diseases.

immunoglobulins. Also known as antibodies and gamma globulins, they're induced by and released in the blood after infections, immunizations and some arthritic diseases, such as lupus erythematosus.

interleukins. Proteins produced by cells of the immune system, such as lympyhocytes. They enhance cell proliferations and functions in immune and inflammatory reactions such as rheumatoid arthritis.

joint. The junction between two or more bones. The most common is the synovial joint, which permits relatively free movement and is most often affected by arthritis. Synovial joints contain a synovial membrane lining on the inside of the joint, which produces nutrients and lubricants for the joint. (*See also* synovial fluid and synovial membrane.)

laminectomy. The surgical removal of part of a vertebra. Usually done to relieve pressure on a spinal nerve caused by a herniated disk or bony spur.

leukocytes. White blood cells. Found in blood and bone marrow, they accumulate in areas of inflammation.

ligament. A band of fibrous tissue that connects bones or cartilages. For example, ligaments that cross joints give strength and stability to those joints.

lymphocyte. A type of white blood cell, normally present in both the bloodstream and lymph tissue, that's involved in immune reactions in most inflammatory and autoimmune diseases, such as rheumatoid arthritis and lupus erythematosus.

macrophage. A type of white blood cell that surrounds and kills microorganisms, removes dead cells and stimulates the action of other immune system cells. Macrophages help destroy bacteria, protozoa and tumor cells. They also release substances that stimulate other cells of the immune system.

magnetic resonance imaging (MRI). A method of imaging tissues of the body using powerful magnets. Cross-sections of soft tissues as well as bone can be depicted.

meniscus (meh-NIS-kus). Menisci (plural) are shock-absorbing cartilages in the knee joint. These crescent-shaped cartilages rest on the top of the shin bone (tibia) and curve around the outer part of the knee (tibial joint surface). They help stabilize the knee and provide cushioning between the thighbone (femur) and shin bone.

myofascial pain. Pain and tenderness in the muscles and adjacent fibrous tissue (fascia). Myofascial pain syndrome (MPS) is a condition characterized by chronic pain in muscle tissues, similar to fibromyalgia. MPS is sometimes the aftermath of injury.

myopathy. Any disease involving muscle. Polymyositis is an example of an inflammatory myopathy that results in muscle weakness.

necrosis. Death of cells or tissue. Necrosis can result when not enough blood is supplied to tissue, whether from injury, radiation or chemicals. Once necrosis occurs, it's not reversible.

neuropathy. Any disease involving nerves. One or more large nerves may be affected (mononeuropathy) or many small peripheral nerves (polyneuropathy).

neutrophils. The most numerous type of white blood cell. Neutrophils help fight bacterial infections.

occupational therapist. A professional trained to help maximize physical potential at home and in the workplace through use of assistive devices and lifestyle adaptations.

omega-3 fatty acids. Polyunsaturated fats that the body can't make and which are derived from food. These fatty acids are beneficial for good health and may also reduce the risks and symptoms for a number of disorders. They appear to exert an anti-inflammatory effect in rheumatoid arthritis. Omega-3 fatty acids are found in fish oil and certain plants.

osteoblasts. Cells that make bone by producing a matrix or frame-work for bone that then becomes mineralized. Bone mass is maintained by a balance between the activity of osteoblasts that form bone and other cells called osteoclasts that break it down.

osteomyelitis. An infection of bone.

osteoporosis. Abnormally reduced bone density. May predispose a person to fractures after slight trauma.

physiatrist. A doctor who specializes in physical medicine and rehabilitation. A physiatrist evaluates and recommends treat-ments that restore function in people with chronic disease.

physical therapist. A trained professional who teaches exercises and other physical activities to aid in rehabilitation and maxi-mize physical ability with less pain.

platelets. Irregular, disc-shaped fragments of bone marrow cells. They are released into the blood where they help prevent bleed-ing by causing blood clots to form. Also called thrombocytes.

polychondritis. An uncommon condition characterized by recur-rent episodes of inflammation of the cartilage structures of the body. Typical areas involved include the nose, ears and wind-pipe (trachea). These tissues may collapse when the cartilage in them is destroyed by the inflammation.

prostaglandins. Hormonelike substances that play a wide range of roles in body functions such as the contraction and relaxation of smooth muscle, the dilation and constriction of blood vessels, and control of blood pressure. They also affect inflammation that occurs in arthritis.

purpura. A reddish-purple skin rash of patches or spots — sometimes raised — which can last from several days to weeks. Most commonly found on the lower extremities and caused by inflamed blood vessels that bleed into tissues beneath the skin. (*See also* vasculitis.)

reflex sympathetic dystrophy. A condition involving the hand or foot and characterized by pain, swelling, coldness and sweating. Also called complex regional pain syndrome.

rheumatic fever. An acute disease involving joints, skin, the heart and other tissues, usually occurring in children, and caused by the body's reaction to a preceding streptococcal infection.

rheumatologist. A doctor who specializes in the diagnosis and treatment of musculoskeletal disorders, including arthritis.

rotator cuff. The tendons of the shoulder muscles that form a sleevelike structure around the joint. Pain and tenderness from injury or inflammation is referred to as rotator cuff syndrome.

sarcoidosis. An inflammatory disease characterized by development of granulomas (small inflammatory nodules) in one or many tissues of the body such as the skin, lungs, liver and spleen. Generally a chronic disease, lasting for several years or longer.

syndesmophyte (sin-DEZ-moe-fyte). A bony outgrowth from a ligament. May cause tenderness and block normal joint movement.

synovectomy. The removal of a synovial membrane from inside a joint such as the knee. May be performed to treat diseases such as rheumatoid arthritis.

synovial fluid. A fluid that lubricates joint surfaces during movement and supplies the joint cartilages with nutrients. Normally, it is viscous and transparent, but with inflammation, it becomes turbid and watery and contains white blood cells.

synovial membrane. The inner lining of synovial joints. (*See also* joint.)

T-Lymphocytes (T-cells). Lymphocytes responsible for cell-mediated immunity in which lymphocytes interact directly with other cells. Two types have been identified — cytotoxic T-lymphocytes and helper T-lymphocytes. When exposed to an antigen, T-lymphocytes divide rapidly and produce large numbers of new T- cells sensitized to that antigen. T-lymphocytes differentiate in the thymus and develop highly specific cell-surface antigen receptors, including some that control the initiation or suppression of cell-mediated immunity. (*See also* lymphocytes.)

tendon. A fibrous cord by which a muscle is attached to a bone or another structure.

tophus. A chalky deposit of urate occurring in gout. Tophi form most often around joints but may occur in other areas, such as ear cartilage.

vasculitis. A condition in which the blood vessels become inflamed. Very small blood vessels can break and cause bleeding into the surrounding tissues, resulting in tiny, reddish-purple spots on the skin known as petechiae (peh-TEEK-ee-ah). Larger spots are called purpura and may look like a bruise. (*See also* purpura.)

whiplash injury. Occurs when the soft tissues of the neck are injured by a sudden jerking or whipping of the head. This type of motion strains the muscles and ligaments of the neck beyond their normal range of motion.

Index

Note: **Boldface blue** page numbers indicate glossary definitions.